T.

Ha...ology

First, second and third edition authors:

Saimah Arif
Arjmand Mufti
James Griffin
Gareth Kitchen

4th Edition

CRASH COURSE

SERIES EDITOR
Dan Horton-Szar
BSc(Hons), MBBS (Hons), MRCGP
Northgate Medical Practice, Canterbury, Kent, UK

FACULTY ADVISORS
Caroline Shiach
BSc(Hons), MBChB, MD, FRCPath, FRCP
Consultant Haematologist, University Department of Haematology, Wythenshawe Hospital, South Manchester University Hospitals NHS Trust, Manchester, UK
Matthew Helbert
MBShB, FRCP, FRCPath, PhD
Consultant Immunologist, Manchester Royal Infirmary, Manchester, UK

Haematology and Immunology

Yousef Gargani
Medical Student
Manchester Medical School
Manchester, UK

MOSBY

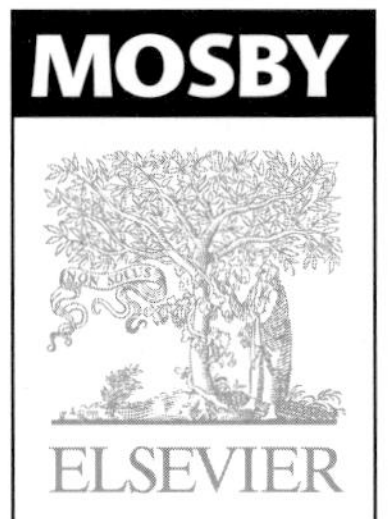

Edinburgh London New York Oxford Philadelphia St Louis Sydney Toronto 2012

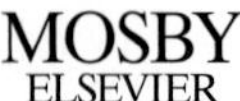

First edition 1998

Second edition 2003

Third edition 2007

Reprinted, 2008, 2010 (twice)

Fourth edition 2012

ISBN: 978 0 7234 3625 6

British Library Cataloguing in Publication Data
A catalogue record for this book is available from the British Library

Library of Congress Cataloging in Publication Data
A catalog record for this book is available from the Library of Congress

Notices

Knowledge and best practice in this field are constantly changing. As new research and experience broaden our understanding, changes in research methods, professional practices, or medical treatment may become necessary.

Practitioners and researchers must always rely on their own experience and knowledge in evaluating and using any information, methods, compounds, or experiments described herein. In using such information or methods they should be mindful of their own safety and the safety of others, including parties for whom they have a professional responsibility.

With respect to any drug or pharmaceutical products identified, readers are advised to check the most current information provided (i) on procedures featured or (ii) by the manufacturer of each product to be administered, to verify the recommended dose or formula, the method and duration of administration, and contraindications. It is the responsibility of practitioners, relying on their own experience and knowledge of their patients, to make diagnoses, to determine dosages and the best treatment for each individual patient, and to take all appropriate safety precautions.

To the fullest extent of the law, neither the Publisher nor the authors, contributors, or editors, assume any liability for any injury and/or damage to persons or property as a matter of products liability, negligence or otherwise, or from any use or operation of any methods, products, instructions, or ideas contained in the material herein.

Commissioning Editor: Jeremy Bowes
Development Editor: Catherine Jackson
Project Manager: Andrew Riley
Designer/Design Direction: Stewart Larking
Illustration Manager: Bruce Hogarth
Icon Illustrations: Geo Parkin

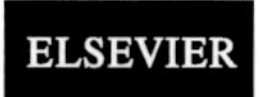

Printed in China

Series editor foreword

The *Crash Course* series first published in 1997 and now, 15 years on, we are still going strong. Medicine never stands still, and the work of keeping this series relevant for today's students is an ongoing process. These fourth editions build on the success of the previous titles and incorporate new and revised material, to keep the series up-to-date with current guidelines for best practice, and recent developments in medical research and pharmacology.

We always listen to feedback from our readers, through focus groups and student reviews of the *Crash Course* titles. For the fourth editions we have completely re-written our self-assessment material to keep up with today's 'single-best answer' and 'extended matching question' formats. The artwork and layout of the titles has also been largely re-worked to make it easier on the eye during long sessions of revision.

Despite fully revising the books with each edition, we hold fast to the principles on which we first developed the series. *Crash Course* will always bring you all the information you need to revise in compact, manageable volumes that integrate basic medical science and clinical practice. The books still maintain the balance between clarity and conciseness, and provide sufficient depth for those aiming at distinction. The authors are medical students and junior doctors who have recent experience of the exams you are now facing, and the accuracy of the material is checked by a team of faculty advisors from across the UK.

I wish you all the best for your future careers!

Dr Dan Horton-Szar

Prefaces

Author

Haematology and immunology are two words that are sure to strike fear into most medical students. They both have the reputation of being complex, lab-based specialities that lose their importance once we reach the 'real world'. In reality, knowledge of both haematology and immunology are immensely important for the practice of all specialities, both clinical and lab-based. This includes topics ranging from anaemia, which is encountered by all clinicians; to non-steroidal anti-inflammatory drugs, which are prescribed by junior doctors throughout the world.

In *Crash Course: Haematology and Immunology* we have made every effort to demonstrate the sound physiological priniciples that underpin the new developments in both specialities. Thus, providing the reader with the foundations needed to grasp the treatments that will emerge after the publication of this book. We have also incorporated clinical scenarios to reinforce the knowledge and understanding of the basic scientific priniciples. We hope you enjoy haematology and immunology.

Yousef Gargani

Faculty advisors

Immunology and haematology are two of the most rapidly moving disciplines in modern medicine. In these two disciplines molecular discoveries are rapidly translated into diagnostic tests and treatments. In this Crash Course you'll read about exciting stuff such as designer drugs for leukaemia and gene therapy for immunodeficiency.

The flip side of all this progress is that these two subjects are not always taught in an up-to-date fashion and some of the newer facts get missed out. It's been a pleasure to work with Yousef on this edition of the book. His charm, intelligence and energy will take him a long way.

Matthew Helbert and Caroline Shiach

Acknowledgements

Figure acknowledgements

Figure 12.7 adapted with permission from C Janeway. Immunobiology, 4th edition. Churchill Livingstone, 1999

Figs. 1.4, 10.5, 10.10, 10.15, 10.18 and 12.11, and Figs 10.20 and 12.20 adapted with permission from I Roitt, D Male and I Brostoff. Immunology, 4th edition. Mosby, 1996

Figs. 2.1, 2.12 and 11.3 taken with permission from A Stevens and J Lowe. Human Histology, 2nd edition. Mosby, 1997

Fig. 1.6 adapted with permission from C Haslett (editor). Davidson's Principles and Practice of Medicine, 18th edition. Churchill Livingstone, 1999

Fig. 5.8 reproduced with permission from M Makris and M Greaves. Blood in Systemic Disease. Mosby, 1997

Fig. 6.17 adapted with permission from T Gordon-Smith and J Marsh. Medicine (Haematology Part 1). The Medicine Publishing Company, 2000

Figs. 2.16, 3.1, 3.7, 3.12, 4.2, 4.6, 4.8, 4.11, 5.9 reproduced with permission from Dacie & Lewis Practical Haematology, 10e, Churchill Livingstone, 2006

Figs. 9.8, 12.2, 12.10, 12.14 reproduced with permission from R Nairn and M Helbert. Immunology for medical students, 2nd edition. Mosby, 2007

Figs. 2.15, 4.4 reproduced with permission from Dr Shiach and the library of Central Manchester University Hospitals

Contents

Principles of haematology

Objectives

You should be able to:

- List the different components that make up blood
- Describe where and how blood cells are generated
- Outline the regulatory factors involved in haemopoiesis
- Relate the structure and function of bone marrow and the spleen
- Discuss disorders involving the spleen.

HINTS AND TIPS

Haematology is the branch of medicine dealing with blood, blood-forming organs and diseases of the blood.

The first part of this book covers haematology and is organized around the various cell types. The production of blood cells, bone marrow and the function of the spleen are discussed in this chapter.

OVERVIEW OF HAEMATOLOGY—THE CELL LINES

All blood cells are derived from a pluripotent stem cell, through a process known as haemopoiesis. These stem cells have two important properties: self-renewal accompanied by proliferation, and differentiation into progenitor cells committed to a specific cell line. Each of the cells produced has an important role which is summarized as follows:

Red blood cells

- **Erythrocytes:** utilize haemoglobin to transport oxygen and carbon dioxide between the lungs and the rest of the body (see Chapter 2).

White blood cells (for immune functions see Chapter 8; for cytological appearance, see Chapter 4)

- **Neutrophils:** phagocytose foreign material or dead/damaged cells at sites of inflammation, activate bactericidal mechanisms and produce mediators of chemotaxis.
- **Eosinophils:** have all the functions of a neutrophil and are important in the host defence against parasites (coated in antibody). They also regulate immediate hypersensitivity reactions.
- **Basophils:** represent the source of most histamine in the human body and can become coated in IgE and release histamine; they mediate type I hypersensitivity reactions. Mast cells in tissues are similar to basophils in blood.
- **Monocytes:** enter tissues to become macrophages. Monocyte-derived cells are found throughout the body as part of the reticuloendothelial system. They phagocytose pathogens and cellular debris and produce various cytokines. They also process and present antigen to lymphocytes as part of the adaptive immune response. Highly specialized mononuclear cells, called dendritic cells, excel in presenting antigen to T cells.
- **B lymphocytes:** as plasma cells they are responsible for immunoglobulin production. They can also become memory B cells.
- **T lymphocytes:** cytotoxic CD8 T cells kill cells infected by intracellular organisms. CD4 T helper cells produce cytokines to activate B cells or macrophages
- **Natural killer (NK) cells:** kill cells they detect as foreign either directly or via antibody-dependent cell-mediated cytotoxicity
- **Platelets:** megakaryocyte fragments involved in the haemostatic response to vascular injury by adhering to subendothelial connective tissue (see Chapter 6).

HINTS AND TIPS

Neutrophils, eosinophils and basophils all have granules in their cytoplasm giving rise to the collective name, granulocytes. Clinicians may use the term granulocyte when only referring to neutrophils, which can cause confusion.

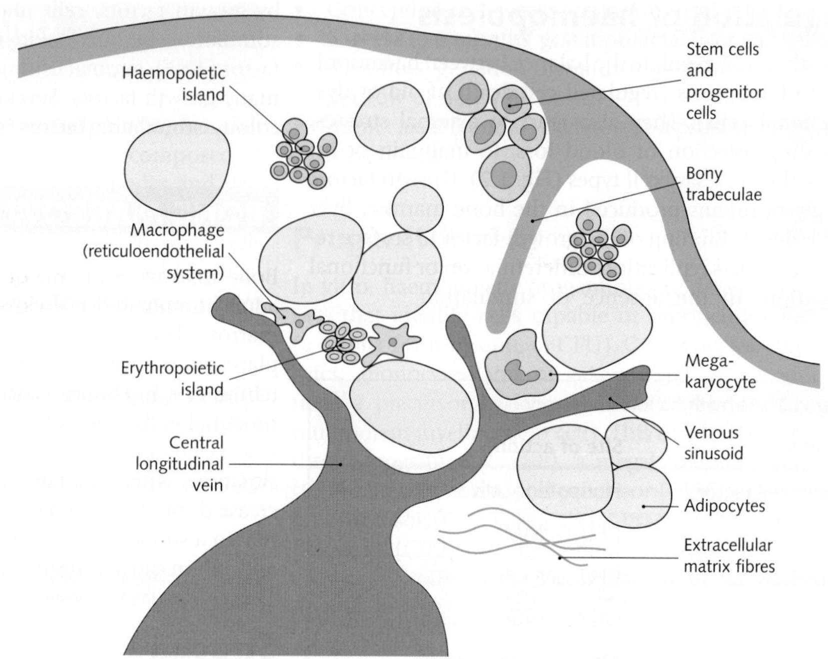

Fig. 1.3 Bone marrow structure. Haemopoietic islands of developing blood cells are interspersed between bony trabeculae and fat cells. A connective tissue stroma of reticular cells and fibres supports the developing cells. Venous plexuses, draining into a central longitudinal vein, transport developed cells out of the bone marrow.

stroma forms specific adhesion contacts with pro-B cells. As B cells develop, they migrate towards the central axis of the marrow cavity and become less dependent on stromal contact. Immature B cells that bind to self cell-surface antigen are removed from the repertoire at this stage. B cells move to the spleen or lymph nodes for final maturation. T lymphocyte precursors leave the bone marrow early in development and are transferred to the thymus for maturation. NK cells accumulate in secondary lymphoid tissue (tonsils, lymph nodes and spleen) prior to activation.

THE SPLEEN

The spleen is a secondary lymphoid organ. It is the site of B and T cell proliferation and of antibody formation, and an important component of the reticuloendothelial system. It is specialized to filter blood, much as the lymph nodes filter lymph, and is a major site of immune response to blood-borne antigens. Blood supply to the spleen is via the splenic artery. Blood is drained via the splenic veins, which join the superior mesenteric vein to form the portal vein.

The spleen is an intraperitoneal organ, normally measuring between 6 and 13 cm; its relations are:

- Anteriorly: the stomach, tail of the pancreas and left colic flexure
- Medially: the left kidney
- Posteriorly: the diaphragm, and ribs 9–11.

Structure

The spleen is surrounded by a dense, irregular, fibroelastic connective tissue capsule that projects fibres, known as trabeculae, into the organ. The two main types of tissue found within the spleen are red pulp and white pulp. These are separated by a marginal zone (Fig. 1.4).

Red pulp

The red pulp is made up of venous sinuses and splenic cords. The splenic cords are composed of reticular fibres. This region predominantly contains erythrocytes but has a large number of macrophages and dendritic cells. The red pulp removes old or defective erythrocytes, white blood cells and platelets from the circulation.

White pulp and marginal zone

The central arteriole is surrounded by a periarteriolar lymphoid sheath (PALS) which predominantly contains T cells. These branch between B cell follicles that

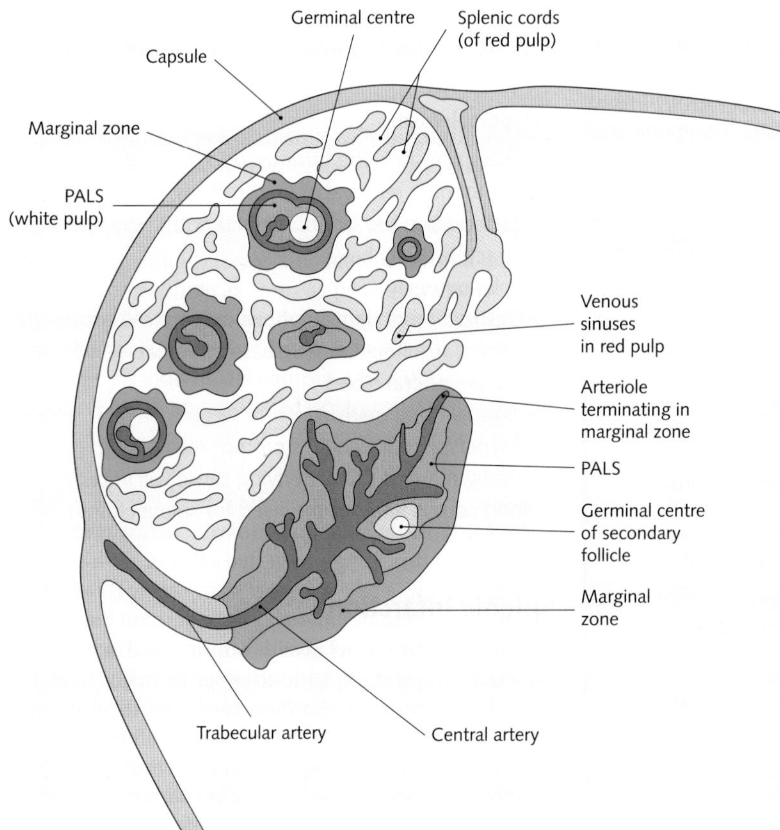

Fig. 1.4 Structure of the spleen. Arterioles entering the spleen are surrounded by T lymphocytes, the periarteriolar lymphoid sheath (PALS). Along with B cells organized into follicles, this constitutes the white pulp.
A germinal centre is a follicle which has been exposed to and reacted to, antigen. These structures are surrounded by a marginal zone containing plasma cells, lymphocytes, macrophages and dendritic cells. The rest of the spleen is composed of splenic cords (red pulp) and venous sinuses.

could be primary (unstimulated) but will be secondary (stimulated) in most patients. The PALS and follicles constitute the white pulp. The white pulp is surrounded by a marginal zone containing plasma cells, T and B lymphocytes, macrophages and dendritic cells. The marginal zone is supplied by venous sinuses that have gaps as wide as 2–3 μm between the endothelial cells. The following functions occur in the marginal zone:

- Antigen-presenting cells sample blood for antigens
- Lymphocytes exit the circulation and migrate to their respective domains
- Monocytes enter the spleen and become macrophages. Here they can attack blood-borne microorganisms
- Lymphocytes and dendritic cells come into contact, allowing initiation of an immune response (see Chapter 10).

The spleen also acts as a reservoir for platelets (20–40% of total pool), erythrocytes (< 5%) and granulocytes (30–50%). If the spleen enlarges for whatever reason it filters more cells, either pooling them or destroying them, thus reducing the amount that are circulating (see Hypersplenism below).

Embryology

The spleen begins as a mesodermal proliferation in the primitive gut during the fifth week of fetal development. It is connected to the body wall by the lienorenal ligament and to the stomach by the gastrolienal ligament.

Disorders of the spleen

HINTS AND TIPS

The spleen must increase significantly in size in order for it to be palpated below the costal margins; thus a palpable splenic edge always indicates splenomegaly.

Red blood cells and haemoglobin 2

Objectives

You should be able to:

- Explain the structure and function of red blood cells
- Outline the process of erythropoiesis, including the functions of erythropoietin
- Discuss iron uptake, transport and excretion
- Describe the structure and function of haemoglobin and be able to interpret dissociation curves
- Summarize the different metabolic pathways active in red blood cells
- Understand and be able to interpret the full blood count and peripheral blood film.

STRUCTURE AND FUNCTION OF ERYTHROCYTES

Erythrocyte structure

Erythrocytes are mature red cells with an average lifespan of 120 days (Fig. 2.1). The normal concentration of erythrocytes in the blood is 3.9–6.5 × 10^{12}/L. Erythrocytes:

- Are not nucleated and contain no organelles
- Contain millions of molecules of haemoglobin, an oxygen-carrying pigment that gives blood its red colour
- Have a characteristic biconcave discoid shape on blood smears. This gives a 20–30% larger surface area than a sphere of the same volume
- Have an average diameter of 7.2 μm
- Are highly flexible and deform readily, allowing passage through vessels of the microvasculature only 3 μm in diameter.

Erythrocyte function

The primary function of erythrocytes is the carriage of oxygen (O_2) and carbon dioxide (CO_2) between the lungs and tissues. The large surface area facilitates this function. They also play an important role in pH buffering.

Gas exchange and transport

The body's resting requirement for O_2 is 250 mL/min. About 200 mL of oxygen is transported in each litre of blood. Multiplied by resting cardiac output (~5 L/min), this means that 1000 mL of O_2 is transported each minute. A small amount of O_2 is dissolved in the blood but the majority is transported by haemoglobin. The oxygen content of the blood depends on three factors:

1. The concentration of haemoglobin
2. The affinity of haemoglobin for oxygen (see p. 17)
3. The solubility of oxygen in the blood (small effect).

CO_2 is carried in the blood in three forms (Fig. 2.2):

1. ~90% as bicarbonate
2. ~5% in the form of carbamino compounds (CO_2 combines with the amino groups of plasma proteins and haemoglobin)
3. ~5% in physical solution (CO_2 is over 20 times more soluble in blood than is O_2).

The large bicarbonate stores of CO_2 are an important pH buffer within the blood. CO_2 levels are tightly regulated by changes in ventilation.

Electrolyte balance

Chloride, potassium and hydrogen ions are transported across the red-cell membrane. One consequence of this is that, in blood stored for transfusion, the extracellular potassium level is quite high due to disruption of active transport. In large transfusions there is potential for hyperkalaemia in some cases.

ERYTHROPOIESIS

Erythropoiesis (Fig. 2.3) is the production of red blood cells from the BFU-GEMM (granulocyte, erythrocyte, monocyte, megakaryocyte) progenitor.

Sequence of erythropoiesis

Erythropoiesis occurs in erythroblastic islands within the bone marrow. These contain macrophages, which supply iron to the surrounding erythroid progenitor cells. The entire sequence (from stem cell to erythrocyte)

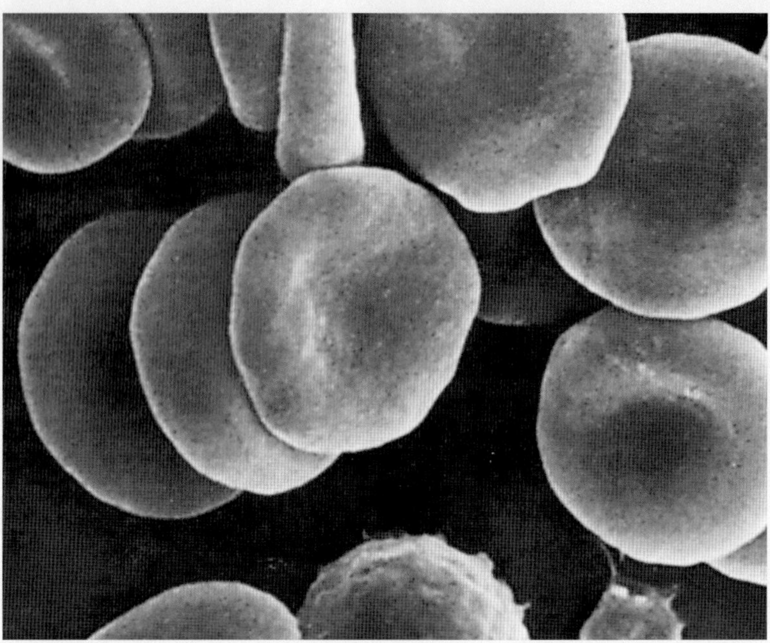

Fig. 2.1 Scanning electron micrograph of red blood cells showing their characteristic discoid, biconcave shape (courtesy of Dr Trevor Gray).

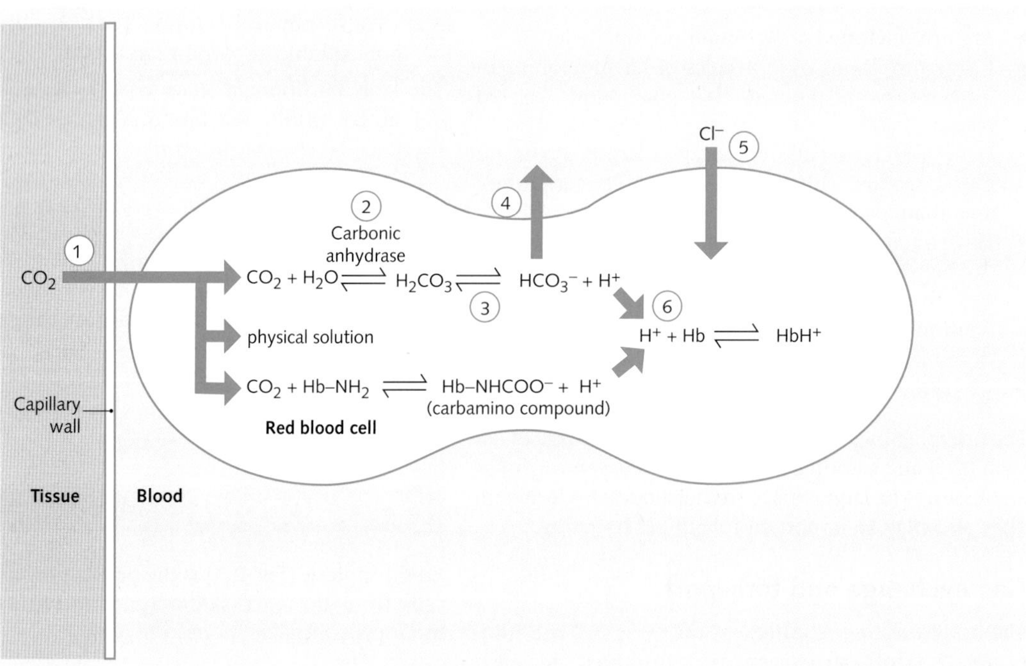

Fig. 2.2 Carbon dioxide (CO_2) transport. CO_2 is transported in both red blood cells and the plasma. Only the intracellular pathways are shown. (1) CO_2 moves along a concentration gradient from tissue to blood. (2) Carbonic anhydrase (not present in plasma) catalyses the formation of carbonic acid (H_2CO_3) from H_2O and CO_2. (3) H_2CO_3 dissociates into protons (H^+) and bicarbonate ions (HCO_3^-). (4) HCO_3^- diffuses along a concentration gradient into the plasma. (5) Chloride ions (Cl^-) enter the cell to maintain electroneutrality, a process known as the 'chloride shift'. (6) H^+, produced as a result of the dissociation of H_2CO_3 and carbamino compounds, is not able to leave the cell. Imidazole groups on the haemoglobin molecule buffer the protons.

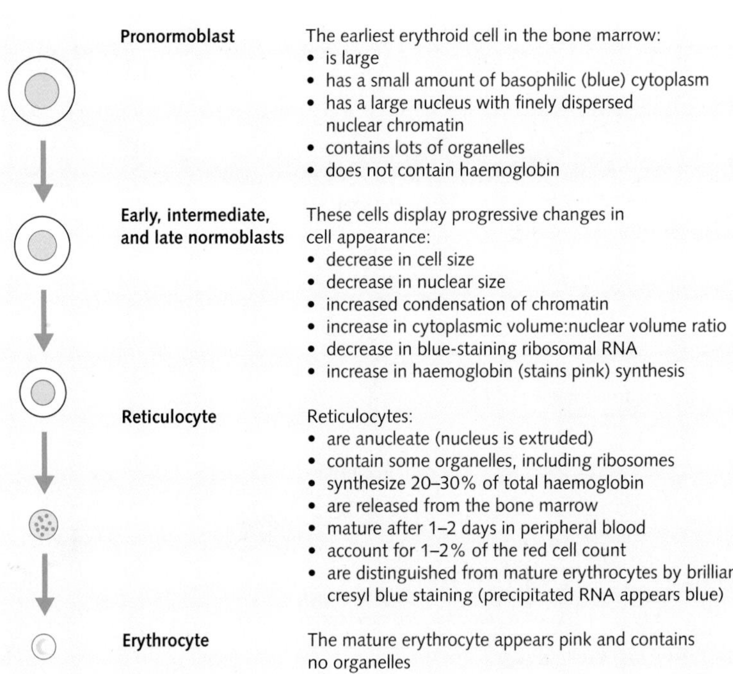

Fig. 2.3 Red cell precursors and the sequence of erythropoiesis. The appearance is that seen with the routine Romanowsky stain, unless otherwise specified.

takes approximately 1 week. Maturation is characterized by the following stages:

- Pronormoblast
- Early, intermediate and late normoblasts
- Reticulocyte
- Erythrocyte.

The production of new blood cells balances the removal of mature cells by the spleen. Following severe erythrocyte depletion, e.g. due to haemolysis, the rate of erythropoiesis in the bone marrow increases. Nucleated precursors and an increased number of reticulocytes will also appear in the peripheral blood.

HINTS AND TIPS

During their maturation, the red cells use their organelles to produce approximately 280 million molecules of haemoglobin. Once they have lost their nucleus and all organelles they become fully matured erythrocytes.

Ineffective erythropoiesis

Each pronormoblast can potentially give rise to 16 erythrocytes, but some normoblasts fail to develop and are phagocytosed by bone marrow macrophages. In a healthy individual, the amount of this 'ineffective erythropoiesis' is small.

Regulation of erythropoiesis

The principal factor regulating erythropoiesis is a hormone called erythropoietin.

Erythropoietin (EPO)

EPO is a heavily glycosylated polypeptide. It is 165 amino acids in length and weighs ≈30,400 kDa. It is secreted by:

- Endothelial cells of the peritubular capillaries in the renal cortex (90%)
- Kupffer cells and hepatocytes in the liver (10%).

Control of erythropoietin drive

The major stimulus for secretion is hypoxia. This can be caused by any factor that gives rise to decreased oxygen transport to tissues relative to tissue demand (Fig. 2.4).

Chronic renal disease (decrease in, or a complete loss of, renal mass) or bilateral nephrectomy will lead to decreased production of EPO, resulting in anaemia. Renal cell carcinomas can produce excess EPO, resulting in an erythrocytosis.

Recombinant EPO, produced in animal cells, may currently be used for:

- Anaemia due to renal failure
- Autologous blood transfusions—to enhance red cell production prior to taking the blood sample

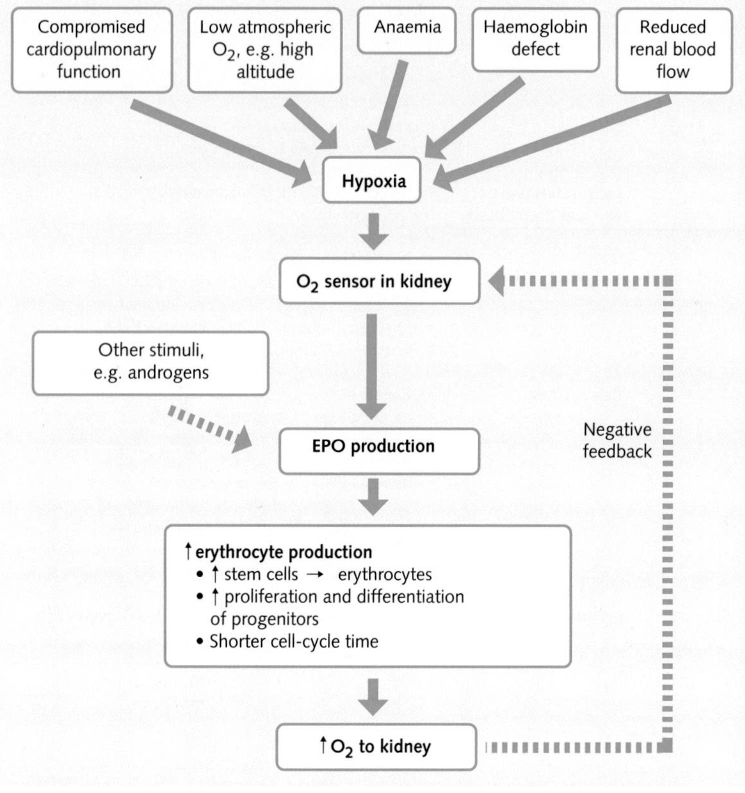

Fig. 2.4 Regulation of erythropoietin (EPO) production. Reduced oxygen (O_2) supply to renal sensors stimulates EPO production. If this is chronically activated, extramedullary erythropoiesis can occur.

- After chemotherapy or bone marrow transplantation
- Anaemia of chronic disease
- Myelodysplastic syndromes. EPO can be combined with G-CSF.

HINTS AND TIPS

Athletes often train at higher altitudes, with lower partial pressures of oxygen, to stimulate erythropoietin (EPO) production and therefore erythropoiesis. This improves their oxygen carrying capacity and, therefore, endurance. Athletes have also been known to use synthetic EPO (illegally) for the same effect.

IRON AND HAEM METABOLISM

Iron metabolism

Uptake and excretion of iron

Iron is found in green vegetables and meats in ferric–protein and haem–protein complexes, respectively. Fortified breakfast cereals are also an important source of iron. Ferric iron is poorly absorbed compared to haem, thus putting vegetarians and vegans at an increased risk of iron deficiency. Consumption of vitamin C with a source of ferric iron aids its absorption, as vitamin C forms complexes with and reduces the ferric iron to ferrous.

Normal uptake and excretion of iron is illustrated in Figure 2.5. The total iron store of the body is around 4 g, mainly as haemoglobin (Fig. 2.6). The daily requirement is normally around 1 mg. Absorption is controlled by proteins in the gut. The rate of iron transfer from epithelial cells to plasma responds to iron requirements, e.g. it is high when stores are low or the rate of erythropoiesis is high.

Iron transport and storage proteins

Free iron is toxic and is, therefore, incorporated into haem or bound to protein within the body. Haem consists of an iron atom at the centre of a protoporphyrin ring. Transferrin transports up to two molecules of iron to tissues that have transferrin receptors, e.g. bone marrow. Both ferritin and haemosiderin store iron in its ferric form. Ferritin is a water-soluble compound, consisting of protein and iron. Haemosiderin is insoluble and consists of aggregates of ferritin that have partially lost their protein component.

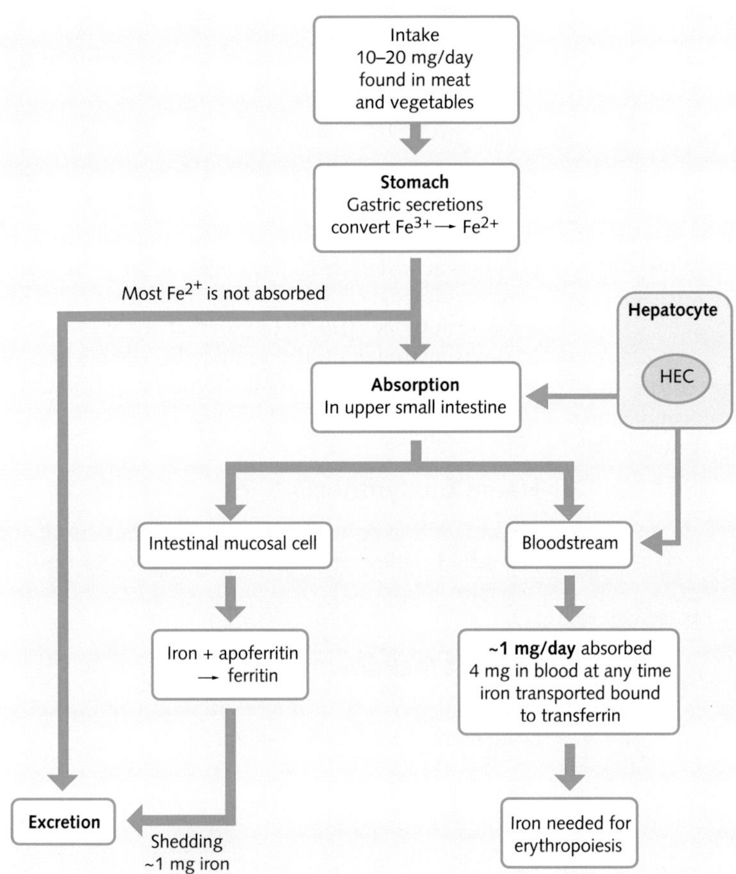

Fig. 2.5 Uptake and excretion of iron. Iron is converted in the stomach from Fe^{3+}, the ferric form to Fe^{2+}, the ferrous form. This process is promoted by ascorbic acid and other reducing agents and inhibited by phytates, tannic acid and tetracycline. Fe^{2+} is actively absorbed in the duodenum and jejunum. Within intestinal mucosal cells, some iron binds apoferritin to form ferritin, a storage compound. The rest is transported, by transferrin in the blood, to storage compartments and the bone marrow. A total of 1 mg of iron is absorbed into the bloodstream each day. Total daily iron turnover is ≈25 mg. Iron in shed mucosal cells or not absorbed from the diet is excreted in the faeces, although a small amount is lost from shed skin cells and excreted in the urine. Extra iron is lost during menstruation (1.5 mg per day compared with 1 mg normally). Hepcidin (HEC) is found predominantly in hepatocytes, although it is also present in plasma. It has a central role in the regulation of iron metabolism and absorption. HEC inhibits absorption as well as the release of iron from macrophages.

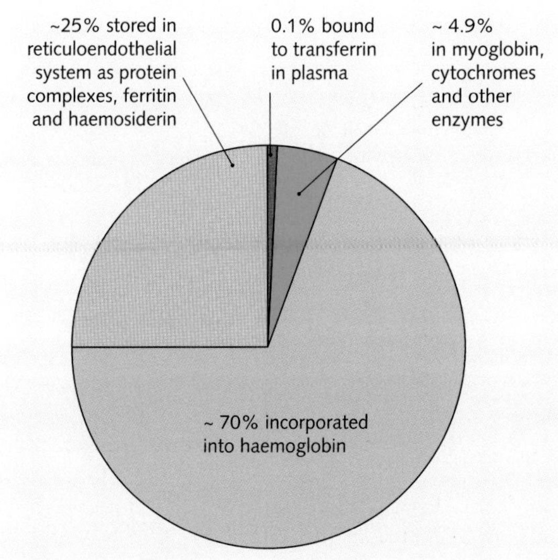

Fig. 2.6 Distribution of iron in the body, totalling ≈4 g.

Iron overload

There is no mechanism for the excretion of excess iron. Consequently, iron overload can occur as a result of:

- Increased absorption
- Parenteral administration.

Excess iron can result in organ damage if it is deposited in the tissues. The heart, liver and endocrine organs are particularly at risk.

Increased absorption

This can be either primary or secondary, and results from the following:

- Primary/hereditary haemochromatosis—an autosomal recessive disorder characterized by excessive intestinal absorption of iron
- Massive ineffective erythropoiesis as seen in thalassaemia syndromes or congenital dyserythropoietic anaemia
- Dietary excess—rare in the developed world but sometimes seen in sub Saharan Africa.

Iatrogenic causes of increased iron uptake

- Multiple blood transfusions (1 unit of blood contains ≈250 mg of iron)
- Inappropriate oral therapy
- Inappropriate parenteral iron therapy.

Treatment

It is important to start therapy as soon as possible to prevent irreversible organ damage. Options include:

- Dietary advice (decrease intake of iron, increase intake of natural chelators)
- Venesection
- Chelation therapy—desferrioxamine is an iron-chelating agent that is administered subcutaneously or intravenously. Two oral chelating agents, deferiprone and deferasirox, are now also licensed for use.

Haemochromatosis

This condition is autosomal recessive. The affected gene, HFE, is located on Chromosome 6. Expression of HFE is required for hepcidin synthesis. Both of the common mutations, C282Y (80%) and H63D (20%) result in decreased levels of hepcidin and increased iron absorption.

Clinical features of presentation after the age of 40 include fatigue, hepatomegaly (which may progress to cirrhosis), bronze skin pigmentation, chondrocalcinosis, pseudogout, diabetes mellitus, hypopituitarism, hypogonadism, cardiac arrhythmias and cardiomyopathy. However there is marked heterogeneity and only about 5% of homozygotes present with symptoms. Men present more commonly than women. Alcohol may promote disease presentation.

Management includes screening first degree relatives, venesection, chelation with desferrioxamine and liver transplant.

Haem metabolism

Haem belongs to a family of compounds known as the porphyrins, which are characterized by the presence of a tetrapyrrole ring. Haem is an iron-containing derivative, the iron ion (Fe^{2+}) being located at the centre of the tetrapyrrole ring of protoporphyrin IX. The haem group is responsible for the oxygen-binding properties of haemoglobin.

Haem biosynthesis

Haem synthesis occurs in the mitochondria of immature red cells in the bone marrow by a process outlined in Figure 2.7.

Haem breakdown

Degradation occurs in the macrophages of the spleen, bone marrow and liver (Fig. 2.8).

HINTS AND TIPS

Bilirubin is a yellow pigment. If haem is broken down faster than the liver can conjugate it, e.g. when haemoglobin is released in haemolytic anaemias, levels of unconjugated bilirubin rise. This bilirubin is then deposited in the dermis resulting in a (pre-hepatic) jaundice.

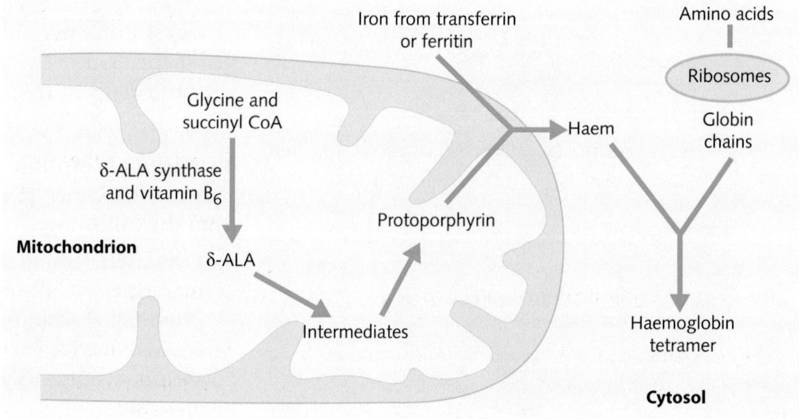

Fig. 2.7 Haem biosynthesis within the immature red cell. Glycine and succinyl coenzyme A (CoA) combine to form δ-aminolaevulinic acid (δ-ALA), a reaction controlled by δ-ALA synthase and the coenzyme vitamin B_6. δ-ALA is converted to protoporphyrin, which combines with ferrous iron to form haem. The haem molecule combines with a globin chain. Haemoglobin is formed by a tetramer of these haem–globin complexes.

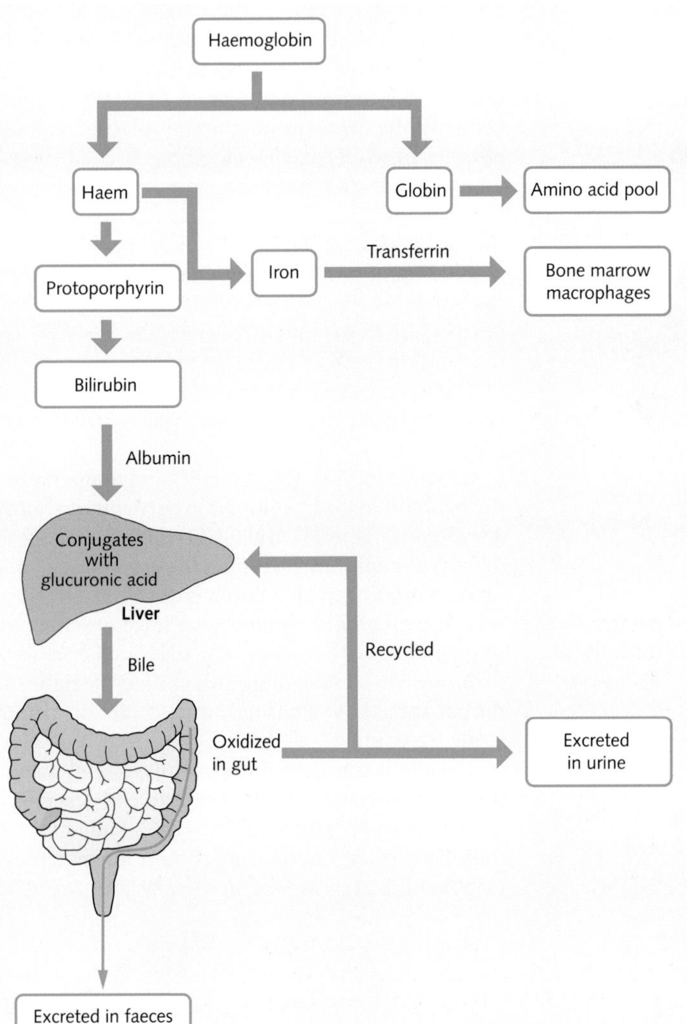

Fig. 2.8 Degradation of haemoglobin. Amino acids from the globin chains are recycled to produce new proteins. Iron is transported by transferrin to the bone marrow to produce new erythrocytes. Protoporphyrin is degraded to bilirubin, which is insoluble and bound to albumin in the blood, described as unconjugated bilirubin, until it reaches the liver where it is conjugated to make it water soluble and excreted in bile. Bilirubin is excreted in the faeces or oxidised to urobilinogen to be reabsorbed and recycled, or excreted in the urine.

HAEMOGLOBIN

Structure of haemoglobin

Haemoglobin is composed of four globin chains held together by non-covalent interactions (Fig. 2.9). Each globin chain has a hydrophobic crevice, or haem pocket, which contains the haem molecule. Each haemoglobin can, therefore, carry 4 molecules of oxygen. The haem pocket allows O_2 binding, while protecting the iron atom from oxidation.

Different types of haemoglobin are present at different stages of development (Fig. 2.10). Adult haemoglobin (HbA) contains two α- and two β-chains, which are arranged as two dimers, written 2(αβ). The globin chains interact with each other in an allosteric fashion, i.e. they bind with each other away from their active sites. The other major haem-containing protein in humans is myoglobin, which consists of a single chain associated with a haem group. It is found principally in muscle, where it provides an oxygen reserve. The four haemoglobin subunits are structurally similar to myoglobin.

The genetics of haemoglobin

The genes encoding the ϵ-, γ-, δ- and β-chains are found on chromosome 11. The ζ- and two copies of the α-chain genes are found on chromosome 16. Each globin gene has three exons separated by two introns. The

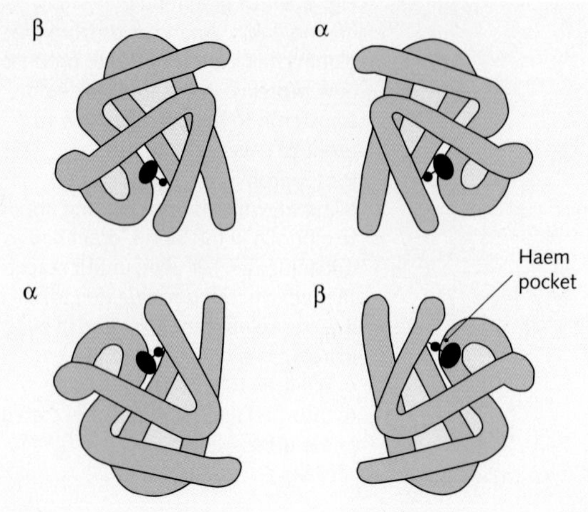

Fig. 2.9 Structure of adult haemoglobin. The α-chain is 141 amino acids long; the β-chain 146 amino acids. A haem pocket can be seen in each globin chain.

different globin chains are synthesized separately and then come together to form a functional Hb molecule.

HINTS AND TIPS

Haem consists of an Fe^{2+} ion at the centre of a protoporphyrin ring. Haemoglobin consists of a haem molecule with four globin chains. Normal adult haemoglobin contains two α- and two β-chains.

Physiological properties of haemoglobin

Each haemoglobin molecule (Hb) can bind four molecules of oxygen, one at each haem site. In terms of oxygenation, Hb can exist in two configurations. When Hb is oxygenated the globin chains are able to move against each other, which will allow O_2 release. This is known as relaxed (R-) Hb. When O_2 is unloaded, the metabolite 2,3-diphosphoglycerate (2,3-DPG) enters the centre of the deoxyhaemoglobin molecule, reducing its affinity for O_2. Deoxyhaemoglobin is characterized by a relatively large number of ionic and hydrogen bonds between the αβ dimers, which restrict the movement of the globin chains. This is known as taut (T-) Hb.

Binding of one O_2 molecule increases the affinity for oxygen at the remaining haem groups. It is this property of Hb which causes the characteristic sigmoidal (S-shaped) dissociation curve.

The oxygen dissociation curve is a plot of partial pressure of oxygen (*x* axis) against oxygen saturation (*y* axis) (Fig. 2.11).

Changes in CO_2, H^+, 2,3-DPG and temperature shift the position of the haemoglobin curve but do not generally alter its shape. H^+ and 2,3-DPG bind to and stabilize deoxyhaemoglobin, favouring the unloading of oxygen. Oxygen binding to myoglobin is not altered by these factors. Haemoglobin variants also have an effect on the oxygen dissociation curve, e.g. sickle-cell haemoglobin shifts the curve to the right. This shift to the right enables the patient to have a normal exercise tolerance in spite of a low Hb count.

Oxygen is transferred from adult to fetal haemoglobin (HbF) because 2,3-DPG binds to HbF less effectively than to adult Hb (HbA), giving HbF a higher O_2 affinity than HbA. This process is important for maternal HbA to offload oxygen to HbF in the placenta.

HINTS AND TIPS

The shift of the oxygen dissociation curve to the right in the presence of increased H^+ concentration is called the Bohr effect. This facilitates increased O_2 release in the tissues, but increased O_2 uptake in the lungs.

Fig. 2.10 Types of haemoglobin present during different stages of development

Developmental stage	Haemoglobin type	Chains	Note
Embryonic	Hb Gower I Hb Gower II Hb Portland	$\zeta_2\varepsilon_2$ $\alpha_2\varepsilon_2$ $\zeta_2\gamma_2$	
Fetal	HbF	$\alpha_2\gamma_2$	Main Hb in later two-thirds of fetal life and in the newborn until approximately 12 weeks of age; higher affinity for O_2 than HbA
Adult	HbA HbA_2	$\alpha_2\beta_2$ $\alpha_2\delta 2$	Principal Hb; 68,000 kDa –2% of adult Hb

Hb, haemoglobin; HbA, adult haemoglobin; HbF, fetal haemoglobin.

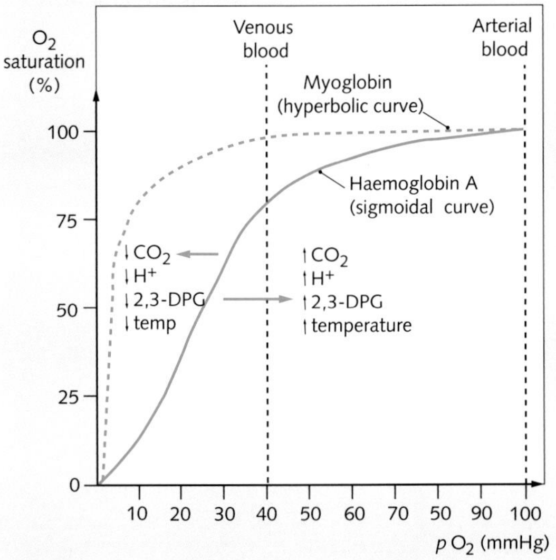

Fig. 2.11 Oxygen dissociation curve for haemoglobin and myoglobin. The haemoglobin curve is sigmoidal in shape because of the cooperative binding of O_2 to haemoglobin. Conversely, unloading of O_2 at one haem group facilitates unloading at the other haem sites. In comparison, the myoglobin curve is hyperbolic in shape, because myoglobin does not release oxygen until the partial pressure of O_2 (pO_2) falls to very low levels. This is because myoglobin does not exhibit cooperative binding. HbA is 100% saturated at a pO_2 of 100 mmHg and 75% saturated at 40 mmHg, the partial pressures of arterial and venous blood, respectively. 2,3-DPG, 2,3-diphosphoglycerate.

THE CYTOSKELETON OF THE RED CELL

Structure

The erythrocyte plasma membrane is supported by a dense, fibrillar, protein shell—the cytoskeleton.

The red-cell cytoskeleton:

- Maintains cell shape and confers strength to the erythrocyte membrane, allowing the cell to withstand the stresses of the circulation
- Permits flexibility, which is important in erythrocyte circulation.

The proteins of the plasma membrane, categorized into integral and peripheral, are important constituents of the cytoskeleton (Fig. 2.12). The band numbers refer to their mobility on electrophoresis.

Integral proteins

Integral proteins penetrate the lipid bilayer of the cell membrane and are closely associated with it. These include band 3 protein and glycophorins.

Peripheral proteins

Peripheral proteins are loosely attached to the lipid bilayer and include spectrin, ankyrin, band 4.1 protein and actin. Dysfunction within the peripheral proteins

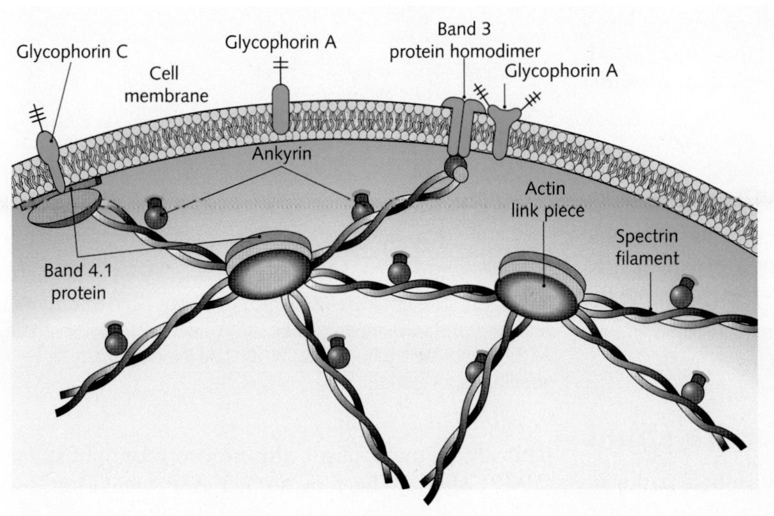

Fig. 2.12 Structure of the red cell cytoskeleton. The hexagonal spectrin lattice is anchored to the membrane by band 3 protein, ankyrin and band 4.1 protein. Spectrin is the primary structural component of the cytoskeleton.

is the basis of some inherited diseases that result in anaemia. The two most common are hereditary spherocytosis and hereditary elliptocytosis (see p. 27).

Surface proteins

There are numerous surface proteins interacting with plasma. Many are linked by the glucosyl phosphatidylinositol (GPI) anchor. Somatic mutation in the gene for phosphatidylinositol glycan protein A (PIG-A) results in the condition paroxysmal nocturnal haemoglobinuria (PNH) (see p. 29).

METABOLISM OF RED CELLS

Glucose is the principal energy source for red cells. It is taken up by facilitated diffusion in an insulin-independent fashion. Because red cells have no mitochondria they cannot metabolize glucose aerobically, therefore it is metabolized via:

- The glycolytic pathway (Embden–Meyerhof pathway)
- The hexose monophosphate shunt.

Glycolysis and the Embden–Meyerhof pathway

This is the glycolytic pathway common to all cells of the human body whereby glucose is metabolized to lactate (Fig. 2.13). There is a net yield of two ATP molecules, but no net NADH production.

$$\text{glucose} + 2P_i + 2ADP \rightarrow 2\ \text{locate} + 2ATP + 2H_2O$$

Defects of glycolytic enzymes are rare. Approximately 95% are associated with pyruvate kinase and are restricted to red blood cells. Insufficient ATP is produced to maintain the structural integrity of the red cell, leading to premature cell death and a haemolytic anaemia (see p. 27).

The Luebering–Rapoport shunt

Only 15–25% of glucose passing through the glycolytic pathway enters this shunt; the function of which is to generate 2,3-diphosphoglycerate (2,3-DPG). Unlike the reaction catalysed by phosphoglycerate kinase, no ATP is produced.

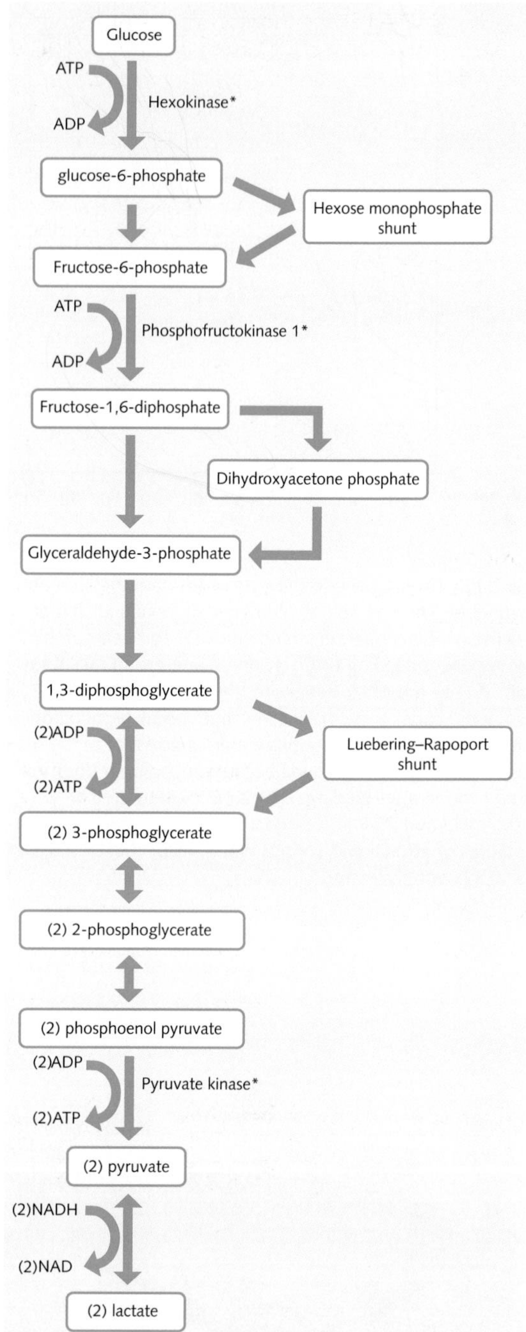

Fig. 2.13 The Embden–Meyerhof pathway. Starred enzymes represent the rate-limiting steps. ADP, adenosine diphosphate; ATP, adenosine triphosphate; NAD/NADH, nicotinamide adenine dinucleotide.

The hexose monophosphate shunt

This is also known as the pentose phosphate pathway. Under normal conditions, 5% of the glucose metabolized by the red cell passes through an oxidative pathway of metabolism, the hexose monophosphate (HMP) shunt. There is no net ATP yield, but two NADPH molecules are produced per molecule of glucose-6-phosphate entering the shunt. The majority of the cell's NADPH is produced in this way. NADPH is important in erythrocytes because it reduces oxidized glutathione (GSSG). Reduced glutathione (GSH) is required to maintain sulphydryl groups in their reduced state, which maintains the integrity of haemoglobin and the cytoskeleton.

Glucose-6-phosphate dehydrogenase deficiency is an X-linked disorder characterized by a lack of the enzyme or by a dysfunctional enzyme (see p. 28). Patients are usually asymptomatic, but oxidant stress can induce acute episodes of haemolysis.

Prevention of haem oxidation

When haemoglobin is oxidized ($Fe^{2+} \rightarrow Fe^{3+}$) it is known as methaemoglobin (metHb). Excess metHb is caused by:

- Toxic substances
- Abnormal haemoglobins resistant to enzymatic reduction (M haemoglobins)
- NADH methaemoglobin reductase deficiency (rare).

The reduced haemoglobin can bind to albumin and has a reduced oxygen-carrying capability. NADH from the Embden-Meyerhof pathway and NADH methaemoglobin reductase are important in ensuring that iron remains in its reduced form.

HINTS AND TIPS

Normal ranges can vary with each laboratory. It is, therefore, important to check the normal ranges of the laboratory from which you are receiving the blood results. The normal range is usually printed close to the result.

FULL BLOOD COUNT AND RETICULOCYTE COUNT

Blood samples are added to ethylenediaminetetraacetic acid (EDTA), an anticoagulant. The samples are tested by an automated analyser, which provides the following information:

- Hb concentration, haematocrit, red-cell count, mean cell volume (MCV), mean cell haemoglobin (MCH) and mean cell haemoglobin concentration (MCHC)
- White-cell count with differential
- Platelet count: some laboratories produce additional parameters
- RDW (red cell distribution width) : a measure of the range of red blood cell size in a sample.

Red-cell parameters and the diagnostic inferences of abnormalities of the full blood count are shown in Figure 2.14. When interpreting results it is important

Fig. 2.14 Red-cell parameters on peripheral full blood count

Parameter	Normal range		Diagnostic inference of abnormalities
	Male	Female	
Red-cell count	4.4–5.8 × 10^{12}/L	4.0–5.2 × 10^{12}/L	
Haemoglobin Packed cell volume or haematocrit	13–17 g/dL 40–51%	12–15 g/dL 38–48%	↑ Polycythaemia ↓ Anaemia
Mean cell volume	80–100 fL		↑ (macrocytic) Vitamin B_{12} or folate deficiency, pregnancy, neonates, alcohol or chronic liver disease (may be haemolysis or aplastic anaemia) ↓ (microcytic) Iron deficiency, thalassaemia or anaemia of chronic disease
Mean cell haemoglobin	27–32 pg		↓ (hypochromic) Occurs with microcytosis
Mean cell haemoglobin concentration	32–36 g/dL		
Reticulocyte count	1–2% of circulating red cells 10–100 × 10^9/L		↑ (reticulocytosis) Haemolytic anaemias and after acute blood loss (reticulocytopenia) Impaired red-cell production

Packed cell volume, otherwise known as the haematocrit, is equal to the red-cell count multiplied by the mean cell volume. Mean cell haemoglobin is the haemoglobin divided by the red-cell count, while the mean cell haemoglobin concentration is the haemoglobin divided by the haematocrit. Automated analysers are increasingly able to carry out reticulocyte counts, although they are also carried out on peripheral blood films stained with new methylene blue. The normal range represents values for 95% of the population (mean ±2 standard deviations).

to remember that normal ranges vary between populations and different laboratories.

PERIPHERAL BLOOD FILM

Examination of a peripheral blood film is a simple haematological investigation, which can provide a significant amount of information. Blood is evenly spread into a film on a glass slide, which is then dried and stained, most often with a Romanowsky stain. The peripheral blood film shows the morphology of blood cells and can show inclusions within the cells.

Normal red blood cells

Normal red cells from peripheral blood films are shown in Figures 2.15 and 2.16.

Abnormalities of red blood cells that are identified on the peripheral blood film are shown in Figure 2.17. Refer back to this figure throughout the following chapters.

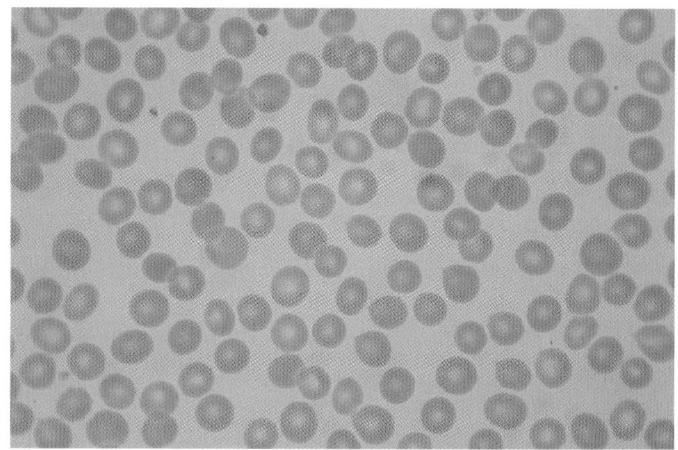

Fig. 2.15 Normal red cells and platelets. Normal red cells are < 7.2 μm in diameter, and have a central pallor due to their biconcave shape. Platelets are seen on the film as small, irregular, densely staining cells.

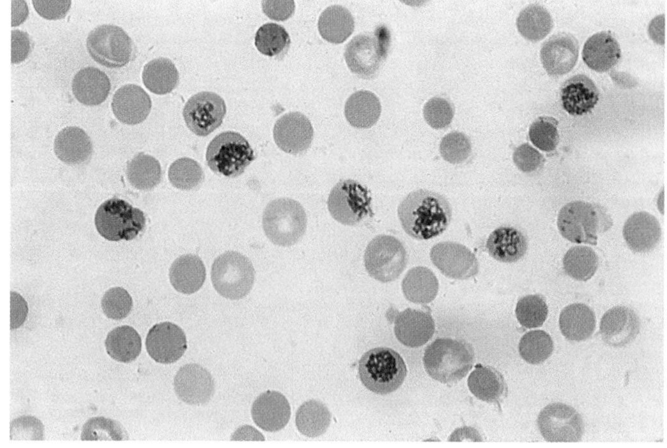

Fig. 2.16 Reticulocytes can be detected using supravital staining, which precipitates RNA in the cell. They are usually present in the blood in small numbers.

Fig. 2.17 Red cell abnorma		
Abnormality	**Desc**	**erences**
Anisocytosis	Incre	micro- and macrocytosis
Poikilocytosis	Incre	s are diagnostic for certain
Spherocytes	Smal	ierocytosis, warm AIHA
Sickle cells	Cres	emia
Target cells	Cells areas	syndromes, sickle-cell on deficiency, liver disease
Teardrop cells	Tear	extramedullary haemopoiesis
Elliptocyte	Elliptical cell	Hereditary elliptocytosis
Echinocyte	Long projections from cell surface	Renal disease
Acanthocyte	Irregular outline	Liver disease, postsplenectomy, abetalipoproteinaemia, pyruvate kinase deficiency
Fragments	Small red cell fragments	DIC, microangiopathy, cardiac valve replacement
Howell–Jolly bodies	Small nuclear inclusions normally removed by the spleen	Postsplenectomy, hyposplenism
Heinz bodies	Precipitates of oxidized denatured haemoglobin	Glucose-6-phosphate dehydrogenase deficiency
Hypochromia	Large area of central pallor	Reduced mean cell haemoglobin (see Figure 2.14)
Polychromasia (recticulocytosis)	Large, bluish cells best seen on supravital staining with new methylene blue	See Figure 2.14
Rouleaux	Red cell stacking (like piles of coins)	Multiple myeloma, Waldenström's macroglobulinaemia, any case with a high ESR

The normal red cell is normochromic, normocytic and has an area of central pallor. AIHA, autoimmune haemolytic anaemia; DIC, disseminated intravascular coagulation; ESR, erythrocyte sedimentation rate.

Red blood cell disorders

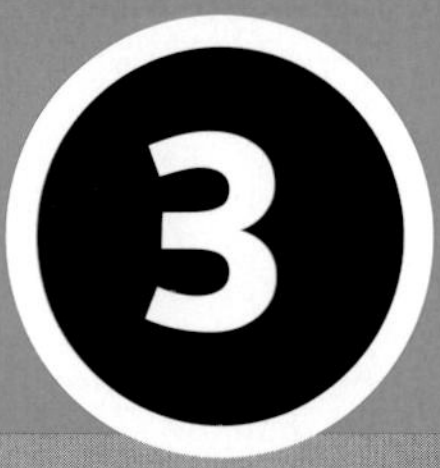

Objectives

You should be able to:

- Demonstrate a good understanding of the different types of anaemia
- Distinguish iron deficiency from anaemia of chronic disease
- Understand the physiology of haemolysis
- Understand the aetiology of sickle cell anaemia and thalassaemia
- Discuss the different forms of polycythaemia.

HINTS AND TIPS

Anaemia is a low level of haemoglobin in the blood. Haemoglobin values of less than 13 g/dL for men and 12 g/dL for women indicate anaemia, although this does not indicate the need for a blood transfusion.

Anaemia is a common problem worldwide, affecting as much as one-third of the world's population. It can be caused by decreased production or increased destruction of erythrocytes, or by blood loss. The causes of anaemia worldwide will reflect local patterns of disease. In the UK the most common cause of anaemia is iron deficiency. In hospitals, however, anaemias secondary to chronic disease predominate. In some developing countries, human immunodeficiency virus (HIV), tuberculosis (TB), hookworm and malaria are the most important causes.

The physiological response to anaemia is an attempt to maintain adequate oxygenation of the body. The level of 2,3-DPG rises to ensure that oxygen is unloaded at the tissues. The cardiac output increases and the circulation becomes hyperdynamic. This can be detected by a rapid pulse and the appearance of heart murmurs. Anaemic patients are often pale. Symptoms vary depending on the cause. They are listed in Figure 3.1, and include:

- Fatigue
- Dyspnoea
- Palpitations
- Headache
- Tinnitus
- Anorexia and bowel disturbance.

Anaemias may be classified either morphologically or by cause. Anaemias are micro-, normo- or macrocytic, depending on the mean cell volume (MCV). The mean amount of haemoglobin in each erythrocyte (MCH) is also measured. If the MCH is low, the anaemia is hypochromic. All of this information is usually given in a full blood count result.

ANAEMIA CAUSED BY HAEMATINIC DEFICIENCY

Iron-deficiency anaemia

Iron deficiency is the most common cause of anaemia worldwide. It occurs most frequently in women of reproductive age. If iron utilization outweighs intake, stores eventually become depleted resulting in anaemia. Causes of iron-deficiency anaemia include:

- Decreased iron intake, e.g. due to poor diet
- Increased iron requirement, e.g. during growth, pregnancy and lactation
- Chronic blood loss, e.g. heavy menstrual bleeding or gastrointestinal (GI) blood loss
- Decreased iron absorption, e.g. after gastrectomy.

HINTS AND TIPS

Iron deficiency in premenopausal women is most commonly caused by menstrual losses. Iron deficiency anaemia in a postmenopausal woman or a man should raise suspicion of a gastrointestinal (GI) bleed, such as a peptic ulcer or an occult GI cancer.

The signs and symptoms of iron-deficiency anaemia (Fig. 3.1) are often only apparent when the haemoglobin level drops below 8 g/dL.

Fig. 3.1 Signs and symptoms of iron-deficiency anaemia

Features common to other anaemias	Features specific to iron deficiency
• Fatigue • Dizziness • Headache • Shortness of breath • Palpitations • Angina • Intermittent claudication • Pallor • Tachycardia • Flow murmur • Congestive cardiac failure	• Glossitis (smooth, sore, red tongue) • Koilonychia (spoon-shaped nails) • Angular stomatitis (sores and cracks at corners of mouth) • Alopecia • Pica (unusual dietary cravings, e.g. for clay and ice)

An atrophic gastritis can also be seen with iron deficiency. In Plummer–Vinson or Paterson–Kelly syndrome, dysphagia and pharyngeal or oesophageal webs accompany the iron-deficiency anaemia.

The haematological findings are:

- A microcytic, hypochromic anaemia (Fig. 3.2)
- Reduced serum iron and ferritin (to distinguish from thalassaemia traits, see p. 31)
- Increased serum transferrin and total iron-binding capacity (TIBC) (to distinguish from anaemia of chronic disease)
- Reduced plasma transferrin saturation
- Absence of iron stores demonstrated on bone-marrow smear.

Clinical management involves identifying and treating the underlying cause of the iron deficiency, as well as supplementation. Oral administration of iron is in the form of ferrous sulphate tablets. This must be continued for 4–6 months to replenish iron stores. Common side effects of oral iron supplementation include constipation, diarrhoea and dark faeces. Parenteral iron is used if the patient has malabsorption or cannot tolerate oral preparations.

ANAEMIA OF CHRONIC DISEASE

This is the most common type of anaemia seen in hospital inpatients and in the elderly (and, therefore, it is important to be able to understand and differentiate). It is associated with chronic conditions such as infections, diabetes, obesity, neoplasms and disorders of the immune system. The mechanism behind anaemia of chronic disease is complex but is thought to relate to activation of cellular immunity and the production of proinflammatory cytokines.

Activated macrophages are erythrophagocytic and secrete cytokines, such as TNF, resulting in decreased erythropoiesis and red cell lifespan. The anaemia is usually normocytic and normochromic, although a microcytic hypochromic anaemia occurs in approximately one-third of cases.

The anaemia responds poorly to iron therapy and is correctable only by treatment of the underlying cause. Erythropoietin (EPO) can help to increase erythrocyte production (but it is rarely used).

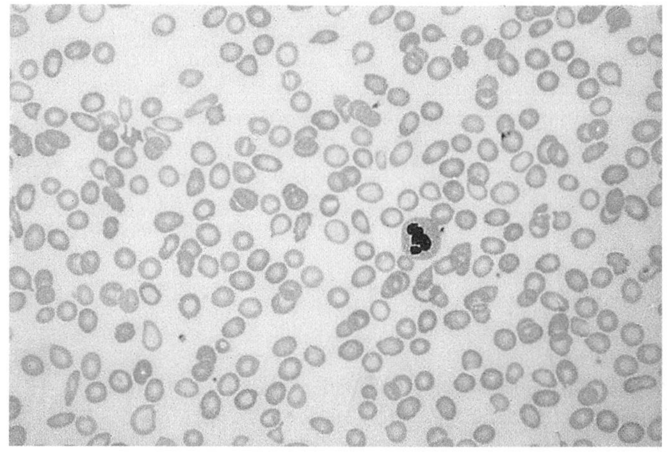

Fig. 3.2 Iron-deficiency anaemia. Red blood cells are typically hypochromic and microcytic.

Making the diagnosis of anaemia of chronic disease or iron-deficiency anaemia

If the MCV is exceptionally low (< 70 fL), iron deficiency is the most likely cause.

The important concept to understand is that in anaemia of chronic disease there is no deficiency of iron, only a deficiency in the ability to utilize iron stores. Therefore, serum iron is low in both conditions.

- Assessment of iron status in iron deficiency:
  - Serum iron: low
  - Ferritin: low
  - Serum transferrin: increased or normal
  - Serum transferrin receptors: increased
- Assessment of iron status in chronic disease:
  - Serum iron: low
  - Ferritin: increased or normal
  - Serum transferrin: decreased or normal
  - Serum transferrin receptors: decreased or normal.

Other important causes of microcytic anaemia are thalassaemia traits. These haemoglobin defects are detailed on page 31.

Other causes of microcytic anaemia that should be considered are:

- Sideroblastic anaemia (which can be hereditary or acquired) is a refractory anaemia characterized by increased bone marrow iron and the presence of ringed sideroblasts (red-cell precursors containing iron granules surrounding the nucleus). Cells in the peripheral blood are hypochromic. Some respond to vitamin B_6, particularly those with the hereditary type. Vitamin B_6 is a cofactor for haem synthesis, and deficiency prevents iron incorporation.
- Lead poisoning, which inhibits both haem and globin synthesis and can also cause abdominal pain and neuropathies.

A summary of the causes of microcytic anaemias is shown in Figure 3.3.

HINTS AND TIPS

Chronic renal failure is almost always associated with anaemia. A decreased renal mass results in reduced production of erythropoietin (EPO). The anaemia is usually normochromic normocytic.

Megaloblastic anaemias

In megaloblastic anaemias, impaired DNA synthesis results in the appearance of megaloblasts (abnormal red cell precursors) in the marrow. Megaloblasts are large cells which contain relatively large abnormal nuclei with finely dispersed chromatin. Anaemia occurs because megaloblasts are removed by bone marrow phagocytes (ineffective erythropoiesis). Megaloblastic anaemia is usually due to deficiency of vitamin B_{12} and/or folate. Both act as coenzymes in the pathway of DNA synthesis. Haematological findings include:

- Macrocytic anaemia (leucopenia and thrombocytopenia in severe megaloblastic anaemia)
- Hypersegmentation of neutrophil nuclei (right shift)
- Megaloblasts seen on bone marrow smear
- Low serum vitamin B_{12} levels or reduced red cell folate content.

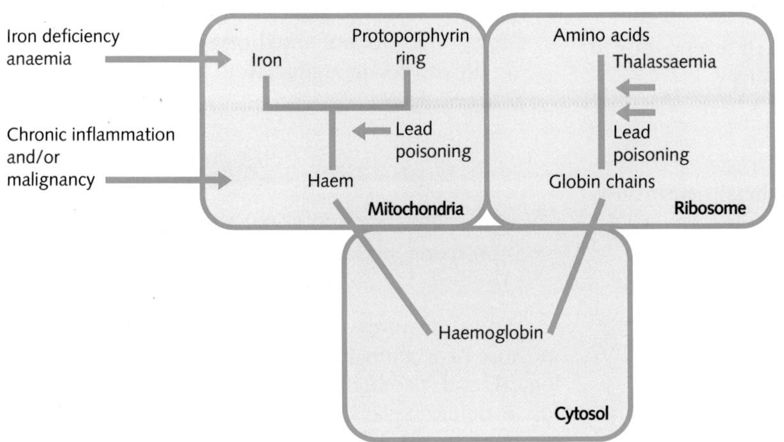

Fig. 3.3 Causes of microcytic anaemia and sites at which haemoglobin production is affected within the developing red cell.

Vitamin B_{12} deficiency

Vitamin B_{12} consists of cobalamin bound to a methyl or adenosyl group. It is found mainly in foods of animal origin (particularly seafood, meat and dairy products) and is not affected by cooking. Intrinsic factor (IF) secreted from gastric parietal cells binds to vitamin B_{12}, protecting it from degradation by stomach acid. Absorption occurs in the terminal ileum. Transport within the body is with the plasma-binding protein transcobalamin II.

Vitamin B_{12} is stored in the liver. Body stores are large (~2–3 mg), and the daily rate of loss in urine and faeces is small relative to daily requirements (1–2 μg); therefore, it takes more than 2 years after the onset of the cause of vitamin B_{12} deficiency for anaemia to develop.

Causes of B_{12} deficiency include:

- Dietary, e.g. due to veganism (rare)
- Intrinsic factor deficiency, e.g. due to pernicious anaemia, postgastrectomy or congenital
- Intestinal malabsorption, e.g. due to diseases of the terminal ileum, such as Crohn's disease
- Blind loop or diverticulae in the small bowel, which breed bacteria that utilize vitamin B_{12}.

Pernicious anaemia

Pernicious anaemia is an autoimmune chronic atrophic gastritis and is the most common cause of vitamin B_{12} deficiency in adults. Autoantibodies directed against both the gastric parietal cells and IF are detectable in the serum and gastric juice of most patients. Damage to the parietal cells results in failure of IF secretion and vitamin B_{12} absorption. Achlorhydria is an accompanying feature (parietal cells are also responsible for secreting H^+). Pernicious anaemia is associated with autoimmune thyroid disease and patients are at increased risk of gastric carcinoma. Presenting patients often have a positive family history of pernicious anaemia and/or thyroid disease.

Clinical features of vitamin B_{12} deficiency include:

- A lemon-yellow colour to the skin (if severe), due to a combination of pallor and jaundice
- Glossitis
- Gastrointestinal disturbances
- Weight loss
- Neurological abnormalities (peripheral neuropathy, subacute combined degeneration of the cord (SCDC) involving the posterior and lateral columns)
- Psychiatric disturbances.

Traditionally the Schilling test was used to diagnose the cause of vitamin B_{12} deficiency, the steps of which are as follows:

1. Oral, radioactively labelled vitamin B_{12} and intramuscular, non-radioactive vitamin B_{12} are administered simultaneously. The intramuscular B_{12} saturates the B_{12}-binding proteins in the plasma and liver, promoting urinary excretion of any absorbed radioactive B_{12}.
2. The urine is collected for 24 hours after B_{12} administration. If less than 10% of the orally administered B_{12} is excreted, absorption of B_{12} is considered impaired.
3. The test is repeated, but this time both oral IF and oral B_{12} are given. If impaired absorption is due to lack of IF (as in pernicious anaemia), B_{12} absorption will be increased. B_{12} absorption will not be increased if the cause of deficiency is malabsorption.

There are now practical issues involving the handling of radioactive materials that make the Schilling test difficult to carry out. Diagnosis is now made from B_{12} levels as well as the presence of autoantibodies to intrinsic factor and parietal cells. Treatment of vitamin B_{12} deficiency is by correction of the underlying cause, if possible, and intramuscular injections of vitamin B_{12} approximately every 3 months.

Folate deficiency

Folates are derived from folic (pteroyl glutamic) acid. They are found in foods, mainly green vegetables and liver, and are destroyed by cooking. Absorption takes place in the duodenum and jejunum. Folate is stored in the liver. Unlike vitamin B_{12}, folate stores are small (10–15 mg) and daily losses are larger relative to daily requirement (100–200 μg), therefore a megaloblastic anaemia develops a few months after the onset of folate deficiency.

Causes of folate deficiency are:

- Decreased intake, e.g. due to poor diet
- Decreased absorption, e.g. due to coeliac disease
- Increased requirement due to rapid cell multiplication, e.g. caused by pregnancy, prematurity, malignancy or haemolytic anaemia
- Increased loss, e.g. due to dialysis
- Drugs, e.g. ethanol, methotrexate (by inhibition of dihydrofolate reductase), trimethoprim and anticonvulsants.

HINTS AND TIPS

Alcohol abuse can cause folate deficiency as a result of malabsorption, malnutrition and increased utilization.

Clinical features of folate deficiency are similar to those of vitamin B_{12} deficiency, without the neurological and psychiatric abnormalities. Treatment of folate deficiency is by correction of any underlying cause and oral supplements of folic acid. Once a megaloblastic anaemia has been diagnosed (i.e. low Hb, high MCV) it is important to refrain from treating folate deficiency without being sure that there is no concurrent vitamin B_{12} deficiency. If there is a possibility of vitamin B_{12} deficiency, supplements should be given at the same time as folic acid to prevent the irreversible and debilitating neurological complications.

HINTS AND TIPS

Red cell folate is low in both vitamin B_{12} and folate deficiency. A serum folate should be used to differentiate between the two.

ANAEMIA DUE TO INCREASED RED-CELL DESTRUCTION (HAEMOLYTIC ANAEMIAS)

In haemolytic anaemias, red cells have a shortened lifespan because they are destroyed at an accelerated rate. This increased red-cell destruction leads to anaemia, which stimulates increased EPO production, leading to compensatory erythropoiesis. The clinical features of haemolytic anaemias result from the increased red-cell destruction and the compensatory increase in red-cell production (Fig. 3.4).

Fig. 3.4 Clinical features of haemolytic anaemias

Cause	Clinical feature	Mechanism
Increased red-cell destruction	Pallor of mucous membranes	↓ Haemoglobin
	Jaundice	↑ Unconjugated serum bilirubin
	Urine darkens on standing	↑ Urobilinogen
	Pigment gallstones	↑ Bilirubin in bile
	Splenomegaly	↑ Red cell destruction
	Absence of plasma haptoglobins	Hb binds haptoglobins; this complex is then removed by macrophages
	Reticulocytosis	Erythrocyte precursors enter the blood
Increased red-cell production	Folate deficiency	Increased erythropoiesis
	Bone deformities	Erythroid hyperplasia causes expansion of marrow cavities

Erythropoiesis can be increased from the normal base-line up to seven-fold, therefore haemolysis may be compensated and not cause anaemia. Increased erythropoiesis results in more reticulocytes being released into the circulation which raises the MCV.

Reduced red cell lifespan can be caused by erythrocyte defects or extracorpuscular defects, as shown in Figure 3.5.

Haemolysis can occur within the circulation or be extravascular:

- **Extravascular haemolysis:** is the route by which red cells are normally broken down and occurs in the macrophages of the spleen, bone marrow and liver.
- **Intravascular haemolysis:** is the destruction of red cells within the circulation. It is characterized by all of the features of extravascular haemolysis (Fig. 3.4), as well as by the following:
  - Haemoglobinaemia: Hb is released into the bloodstream
  - Absence of plasma haptoglobins: normally, free Hb binds haptoglobin to form a complex that is removed by macrophages in the reticuloendothelial system. Thus, intravascular haemolysis normally results in the removal of more haptoglobins
  - Haemoglobinuria: the Hb concentration exceeds the tubular reabsorptive capacity and Hb is therefore excreted in the urine
  - Haemosiderinuria: free Hb is absorbed by proximal tubule cells of the kidney resulting in intracellular deposits of haemosiderin; these are shed in the urine
  - Methaemalbuminaemia: some of the Hb is oxidized and binds to albumin.

Hereditary red-cell defects

The defect is usually intrinsic to the red cell, and morphological abnormalities can often be detected on inspection of a peripheral blood smear.

Cytoskeleton defects

Hereditary spherocytosis

Hereditary spherocytosis is a common autosomal dominant disorder of variable penetrance (prevalence of 1 in 2000 in people of Northern European descent). A defective cytoskeletal protein, most commonly spectrin, causes loss of the membrane. This defect results in progressive spherocytosis and reduced deformability of red cells, leading to extravascular haemolysis (see Fig. 3.6).

Haematological findings include:

- Spherocytes on the peripheral blood smear (Fig. 3.7)
- Increased osmotic fragility: when suspended in saline solutions of varying concentrations, spherocytes lyse in less hypotonic solutions than do normal red cells.

Fig. 3.5 Classification of haemolytic anaemias

Erythrocyte defects		**Extracorpuscular defects**	
Membrane	Hereditary spherocytosis. Hereditary elliptocytosis. Paroxysmal nocturnal haemoglobinuria	Immune	Incompatible transfusions Autoimmune haemolytic anaemia Drug associated
Enzyme	G6PD deficiency PK deficiency	Infection	Malaria Septicaemia
Haemoglobin	Sickle-cell syndromes. Thalassaemia	Drugs/chemicals Mechanical Hypersplenism	Dapsone, sulfasalazine Microangiopathic haemolysis Prosthetic heart valves DIC, HUS, TTP Following long marches Myelofibrosis

DIC, disseminated intravascular coagulation; G6PD, glucose-6-phosphate dehydrogenase; HUS, haemolytic uraemic syndrome; PK, pyruvate kinase; TTP, thrombotic thrombocytopenic purpura.

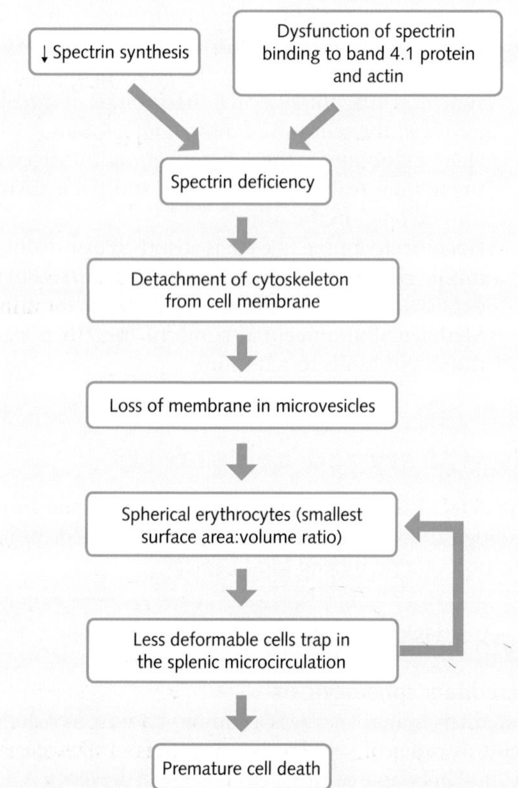

Fig. 3.6 Mechanism of spherocytosis and premature cell death in hereditary spherocytosis due to spectrin deficiency.

The person can be asymptomatic or haemolysis can be present at birth with significant jaundice and anaemia. The usual course after infancy is a low-grade anaemia with intermittent 'crises'. Splenectomy can be used to prevent crises and will result in a rise in the Hb level.

Hereditary elliptocytosis

This autosomal dominant disorder is also due to abnormalities of the cytoskeletal proteins and is most commonly caused by failure of spectrin dimers to form tetramers. It is clinically similar to, but milder than, hereditary spherocytosis. A high proportion of elliptical red cells are seen on the peripheral blood film.

Enzyme defects

Pyruvate kinase deficiency

This is a rare autosomal recessive condition affecting the glycolytic pathway, which results in a lack of ATP production. Erythrocytes become rigid and are destroyed. The blood film shows a poikilocytosis and distorted 'prickle' cells (known as acanthocytes, also seen post-splenectomy). Splenectomy might improve, but not cure, severe anaemias. Like sickle-cell anaemia, patients with pyruvate kinase deficiency can tolerate very low Hb levels due to their oxygen dissociation curve shifting to the right.

Glucose-6-phosphate dehydrogenase deficiency

Glucose-6-phosphate dehydrogenase (G6PD) deficiency is an X-linked disorder affecting the hexose monophosphate shunt (Fig. 3.8). There are over 400 variants of G6PD, two of which account for the vast majority of cases: the African and Mediterranean types. Of these two, the Mediterranean type is clinically more severe, because of a much greater reduction in enzyme function. Patients are generally asymptomatic until haemolysis is precipitated by oxidizing factors such as:

- Infection
- Acidosis, e.g. diabetic ketoacidosis
- Drugs, e.g. primaquine, sulphonamides
- Fava beans ('favism'—only in the Mediterranean type).

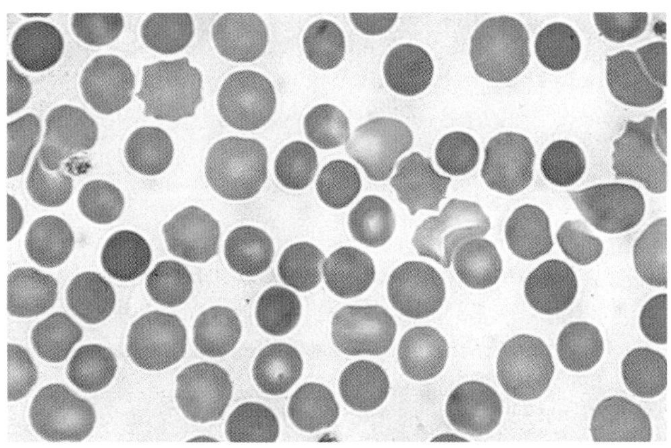

Fig. 3.7 Hereditary spherocytosis. Spherocytes are smaller and thicker than normal red cells but only totally spherical in extreme cases.

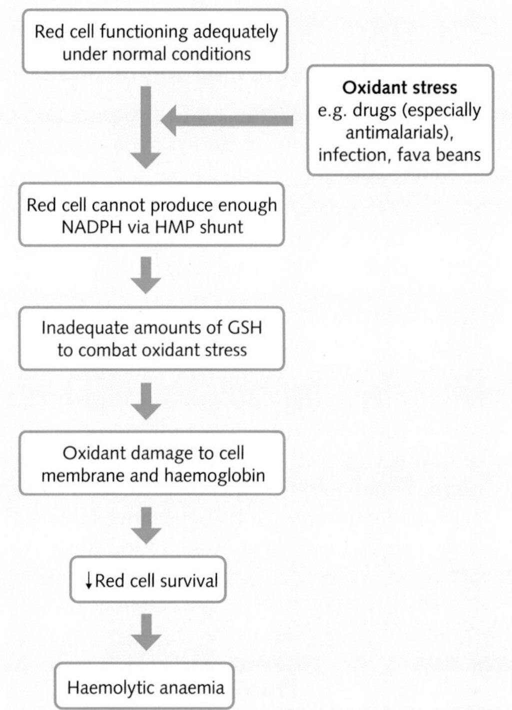

Fig. 3.8 Mechanism of haemolysis in glucose-6-phosphate dehydrogenase deficiency. GSH, reduced glutathione; HMP, hexose monophosphate; NADPH, nicotinamide adenine dinucleotide phosphate.

Haemolysis is primarily intravascular. During a haemolytic crisis, Heinz bodies (precipitates of oxidized, denatured Hb) are generated within red blood cells. Cells that have had Heinz bodies removed upon passing through the spleen, termed 'bite' or 'blister' cells, are seen on the peripheral blood film. Heinz bodies will be seen in patients following splenectomy.

In an asymptomatic patient, the peripheral blood film might be normal. However, G6PD levels are decreased in affected males and carrier females. Assay can be unreliable during or immediately after a haemolytic crisis because reticulocytes (increased in number during a crisis) have higher enzyme levels than mature red cells. In an acute crisis, the precipitating factor should be eliminated and the circulation supported; however, there is no specific treatment.

Other enzyme defects

Several other defects have been identified in enzymes involved in erythrocyte metabolism. They are rare and include hexokinase and glutathione synthetase.

Acquired defects of the red cell

Paroxysmal nocturnal haemoglobinuria (PNH)

This is a rare, acquired red-cell membrane defect. A mutation in the gene coding for phosphatidylinositol glycan protein A (PIG-A) leads to a lack of glycosyl phosphatidylinositol (GPI). GPI anchors certain proteins to the cell membrane. These proteins usually prevent lysis of blood cells by complement (a component of the innate immune system, p. 88) and their absence leads to chronic intravascular haemolysis. PNH is a stem cell disorder, so patients may have leucopenia and thrombocytopenia in addition to anaemia.

Antibody-mediated red-cell destruction

Autoimmune haemolytic anaemias

In the autoimmune haemolytic anaemias (AIHAs), red-cell autoantibodies cause haemolysis. A positive direct

Coombs test can be demonstrated. There are three types of AIHA:

1. Warm AIHA (occurs at body temperature)
2. Cold AIHA (usually occurs below room temperature)
3. Paroxysmal cold haemoglobinuria.

Warm AIHA can be idiopathic or secondary to autoimmune disease (especially systemic lupus erythematosus (SLE)), leukaemias (especially chronic lymphocytic leukaemia), lymphomas and drugs (e.g. mefenamic acid). The clinical features are as follows:

- Anaemia
- Jaundice
- Splenomegaly (almost always, although often very mild)
- Evans' syndrome, which is the combination of warm AIHA and idiopathic thrombocytopenic purpura (ITP) (very rare).

Identified causes should be eliminated. Patients generally respond well to steroids but other immunosuppressive therapies (e.g. azothiaprine), the monoclonal anti-B-cell antibody rituximab or splenectomy might also be required.

Cold AIHA can be idiopathic or secondary to lymphoma, leukaemia or infection (e.g. mycoplasma pneumonia, Epstein–Barr virus). The clinical features are as follows:

- Symptoms worse in cold weather
- Acrocyanosis (purplish discolouration of the skin) due to vascular sludging arising from red-cell agglutination
- Raynaud's phenomenon.

Treatment involves the elimination of any cause and keeping the patient warm. The monoclonal antibody rituximab (anti-CD20) has been shown to be effective in idiopathic cold AIHA and cold AIHA associated with B-lymphoproliferative diseases.

Paroxysmal cold haemoglobinuria is a subset of cold AIHA in which haemolysis occurs at higher temperatures but antibody binding occurs at cold temperatures. This usually presents in children after a viral infection.

The laboratory features of warm and cold AIHAs are compared in Figure 3.9.

Alloimmune haemolytic anaemias

Alloimmune haemolytic anaemias are caused by a reaction between antibodies and blood cells from different people. This occurs following:

- Transfusion of ABO-incompatible blood
- Transfer of maternal antibodies across the placenta in haemolytic disease of the newborn
- Allogeneic transplantation.

Drug-induced immune haemolytic anaemias

Certain drugs (e.g. penicillin, cephalosporins and fludarabine) can precipitate haemolysis via a variety of immune mechanisms.

Other causes of haemolysis

- Mechanical trauma:
  - Classically with mechanical heart valves
  - Microangiopathic haemolytic anaemia occurs when fibrin is deposited in small vessels. This is seen in haemolytic uraemic syndrome, thrombotic thrombocytopenic purpura, disseminated carcinoma, malignant hypertension and Gram-negative septicaemia. It is characterized by red cell fragments (schistocytes) in the blood film

Fig. 3.9 Comparison of laboratory features of autoimmune haemolytic anaemias (AIHAs)

Feature	Warm AIHA	Cold AIHA	Paroxysmal cold haemoglobinuria
Antibody class	IgG	IgM	IgG (Donath-Landsteiner)
Antibody specificity	May be Rhesus	May be I or i antigens	Red cell P antigen
Antibody binding temperature	37 °C	< 32 °C	< 32 °C
Red cell agglutination	x	✓	✓
Complement fixation	**x**	✓	✓
Mechanism of cell destruction	Mainly extravascular	Mainly intravascular	Mainly intravascular
Direct Coombs test	Positive for IgG and complement	Positive for complement	Positive for IgG and complement

- March haemoglobinuria is caused by damage to red cells in the feet during long periods of walking or running. The blood film does not show fragments
- Chemicals and toxins, e.g. lead poisoning, some snake venoms
- Infection, e.g. malaria
- Burns.

HAEMOGLOBINOPATHIES

Thalassaemias

HINTS AND TIPS

In thalassaemias, the inheritance of defective genes encoding for the α- or β-globin chains results in their reduced production.

β-Thalassaemia occurs most commonly in Mediterranean countries, South-East Asia and Africa. There is a partial or complete failure of β-globin chain production.

The abnormal β-chain genes are denoted β^+ and β^0 for partial or complete deficiency, respectively. Severity of disease depends on which abnormal genes have been inherited and whether the individual is heterozygous or homozygous.

α-Thalassaemia is most common in South-East Asia and West Africa. There is a deletion of one, two, three or all four α-globin chain genes. The number of deleted genes relates to the severity of disease, although deletion of all four α-globin chains is incompatible with life.

Deficiency of one globin chain results in the compensatory production of the other to form the Hb molecule. An excess of α-chains (in β-thalassaemia) or β-chains (in α-thalassaemia) results in abnormal aggregation within red-cell precursors, predisposing them to phagocytosis by bone marrow macrophages. Any abnormal red cells that reach the circulation have a shortened lifespan. A number of clinical syndromes are recognized, based on the severity of the anaemia (Fig. 3.10).

β-Thalassaemia major

In β-thalassaemia major, homozygosity for defective genes causes β-chain production to be severely reduced. Investigation reveals:

- Microcytic hypochromic anaemia (Hb 2–3 g/dL) and reticulocytosis (at 6–9 months if not transfused)

Fig. 3.10 Thalassaemia syndromes

Clinical syndrome	Type	Presentation
β-thalassaemia major (Mediterranean or Cooley's anaemia)	Homozygous ($\beta^0\beta^0$, $\beta^+\beta^+$ or $\beta^+\beta^0$)	Onset at 6–9 months; severe anaemia, jaundice, failure to thrive, hepatosplenomegaly, bony abnormalities, gallstones, leg ulcers, intercurrent infections
β-thalassaemia intermedia	A variety of genotypes	Presents at 1–2 years of age with a moderate anaemia
β-thalassaemia minor (trait)	Heterozygous ($\beta^0\beta$ or $\beta^+\beta$)	Usually asymptomatic; mild microcytic hypochromic anaemia (Hb 10–11 g/dL) Raised HbA_2 (4–8% of total Hb, normally 2%)
α-thalassaemia silent carrier	3 α genes present	Usually asymptomatic with no detected abnormalities
α-thalassaemia trait	2 α genes present	Normal or slightly low haemoglobin level with microcytic red cells, usually asymptomatic
HbH disease	1 α gene present	Anaemia (7–11 g/dL); HbH is formed (β_4) Clinical features of chronic haemolysis
Hydrops fetalis	No α genes present	Fetus usually dies in utero Tetramers of γ-chains form a haemoglobin variant, Hb Barts hydrops Prenatal diagnosis with aggressive transfusions in utero can prevent fetal death

Hb, haemoglobin; HbA, adult haemoglobin; HbF, fetal haemoglobin.

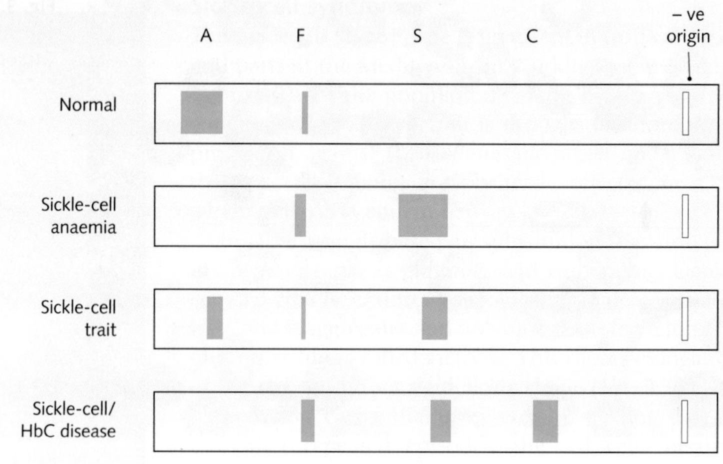

Fig. 3.14 Haemoglobin electrophoresis is used to detect different forms of haemoglobin (Hb). It can detect HbS (sickle haemoglobin), HbC, HbF (fetal haemoglobin), HbA (adult haemoglobin) and HbH (β tetramer, sometimes represented as β_4).

which each of the molecules travels at a different rate, depending on its electrical charge and size. In terms of haemoglobinopathies, the different types of haemoglobin have different structures and, therefore, different weights/charges, so the pattern of bands produced by electrophoresis is different (Fig. 3.14).

ANAEMIA DUE TO BLOOD LOSS

Acute blood loss

Causes of acute blood loss include trauma, surgery, peripartum haemorrhage, haematemesis and haemoptysis. Plasma volume is replaced within 1–3 days of the acute blood loss but it can take several weeks for the red cell mass, and, therefore, haemoglobin, to be replenished. Haematological findings in acute blood loss include:

- A normocytic, normochromic anaemia
- A reticulocytosis that peaks 1–2 weeks after the haemorrhage
- An increase in the number of platelets and neutrophils
- Neutrophil precursors in the peripheral blood.

Red-cell parameters might be normal before compensation for the loss of intravascular volume as both plasma and red cells have been lost in their normal proportions.

Chronic blood loss

The most common causes of chronic blood loss are gastrointestinal lesions and menorrhagia. The consequences are those of iron-deficiency anaemia (see p. 23).

MARROW DEFECTS

Aplastic anaemia

Aplastic anaemia is characterized by pancytopenia and aplasia (hypocellularity) of the bone marrow. There is a reduction in the number of bone-marrow stem cells and those that remain are defective and cannot repopulate the marrow. Causes of aplastic anaemia are listed in Figure 3.15. Treatment is supportive with removal of any causative factors. Specific treatment is with antithymocyte globulin, ciclosporin, haemopoietic growth factors, androgens or stem cell transplantation.

Pure red-cell aplasia

This is a rare condition in which only the red-cell precursors in the bone marrow are defective. Parvovirus B19 causes transient red-cell aplasia.

Fig. 3.15 Causes of aplastic anaemia

Congenital	Acquired
Fanconi type—a rare autosomal recessive condition associated with other congenital anomalies and increased incidence of malignancy	• Idiopathic (50% of cases) • Drugs that cause marrow suppression (e.g. busulphan, chloramphenicol) • Ionizing radiation • Chemicals, e.g. benzene, insecticides • Infection, e.g. viral hepatitis • Paroxysmal nocturnal haemoglobinuria

Other forms of marrow failure

Space-occupying lesions can cause anaemia, e.g. metastatic carcinoma in the bone marrow, which destroys the bone marrow architecture.

Myelodysplasia (see p. 47) may initially present as a macrocytic anaemia.

POLYCYTHAEMIA (ERYTHROCYTOSIS)

Polycythaemia may be primary or secondary. Primary polycythaemia has no physiological benefit and arises from an abnormal clone of cells (p. 46). Secondary polycythaemia occurs as a result of a physiological adaptation to hypoxia, with the erythrocytosis increasing the oxygen-carrying capacity of blood. A summary of the causes of polycythaemia is shown in Figure 3.16.

Apparent polycythaemia can occur as a result of a reduction in the total plasma volume. Investigation to exclude this involves measuring total red cell volume (using ^{51}Cr) and total plasma volume (using ^{123}I-albumin).

HINTS AND TIPS

Venesection, as treatment for secondary polycythaemia, should not aim to drastically reduce the packed cell volume (PCV) as this negates the adaptive advantage of the compensatory erythropoiesis. Treatment should be to a level which reduces the symptoms caused by hyperviscosity (PCV approximately 0.55).

Fig. 3.16 Causes of polycythaemia

Absolute	Relative
Primary • Polycythaemia rubra vera (see p. 46.) Secondary Appropriately increased erythropoietin: • High altitude • Chronic lung disease • Cyanotic heart diseases • Haemoglobin with abnormally high O_2 affinity Inappropriately increased erythropoietin: • Renal disease (carcinoma, cysts, transplants) • Hepatocellular carcinoma • Cerebellar haemangioblastoma • Massive uterine fibroids	Fluid depletion • Dehydration (diarrhoea and vomiting) • Plasma loss, e.g. burns • Diuretic therapy Cigarette smoking Stress (associated with smoking, alcohol, hypertension, obesity)

White blood cells

Objectives

You should be able to:

- Explain the structure of the different classes of white blood cells, and how eac specialized functions
- Discuss the mechanisms involved in leucocytosis
- Describe the causes and features of leucopenia.

STRUCTURE AND FUNCTION OF THE WHITE BLOOD CELLS

See Chapter 9 for a discussion of the immunological functions of white blood cells.

Lymphocytes

Appearance and structure

Lymphocytes (Figs 4.1 and 4.2) are the smallest white cells, measuring 6–15 μm in diameter. In blood they are round but they can change shape outside the circulation. They have round, densely staining, acentric nuclei. The sparse cytoplasm may contain a few lysosome-like granules. Once activated, the amount of cytoplasm increases. B cells and natural killer (NK) cells tend to be larger than T cells. The cells are differentiated by the presence of differing surface markers.

Location

Lymphocytes circulate between tissue, lymphatics and the blood. The lifespan of lymphocytes varies depending on their interaction with antigens. Memory cells can survive for decades.

Function

Lymphocytes in the blood are simply in transit between the bone marrow and lymphoid tissues, which is where they function. They produce antibodies and kill foreign or virally altered cells.

Neutrophils

Appearance and structure

Neutrophils (Figs 4.3 and 4.4), also known as polymorphonuclear leucocytes, measure 9–15 μm in diameter. They have distinctive nuclei containing 2–5 lobes connected by thin chromati cleus has a 'drumstick' apper vated X chromosome. Neutr and large stores of glycogen

Location

Neutrophils circulate in b sponse to chemotactic ag where they survive for 1

Function

Neutrophils are the first tion and, once defunct, pus. They destroy micr release of hydrolytic e

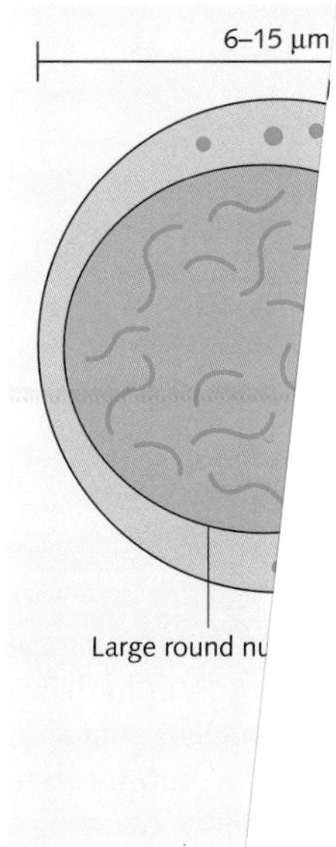

Fig. 4.1 Lymph

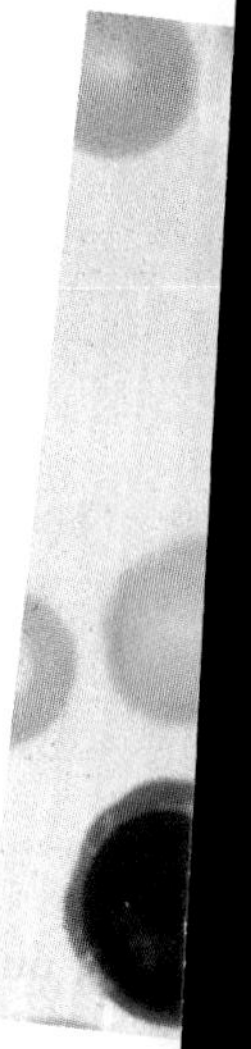

Fig. 4.2 N diameter). T azurophilic

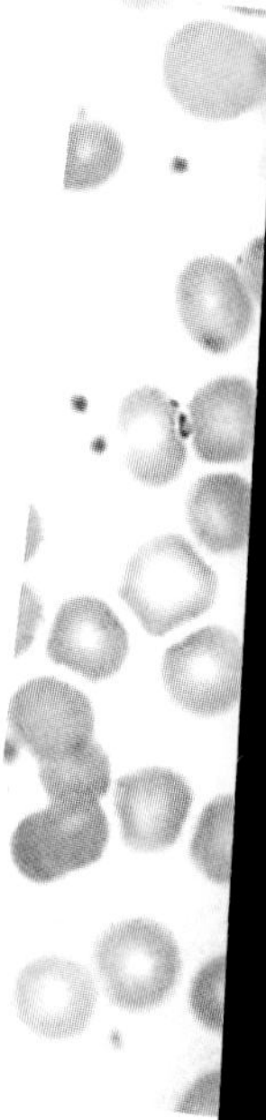

Fig. 4.3 Neutr

Monocyt

Appearance

Monocytes (Fi circulating bloo eter. They have are often prese appearance. Th and vacuole-li appearance. Mi

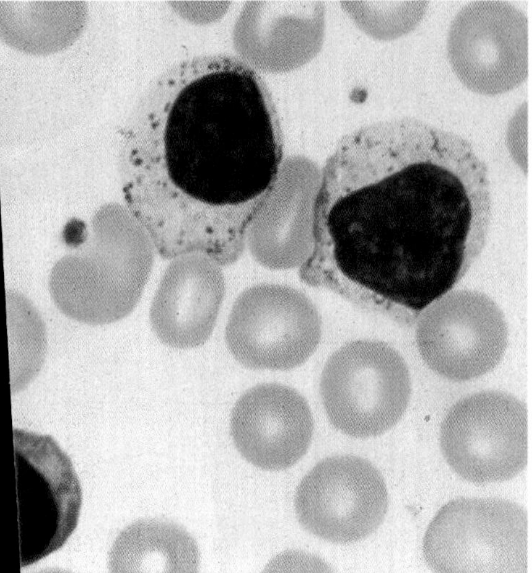

ormal lymphocytes are quite small (on average 9 μm They contain very little cytoplasm and occasional granules.

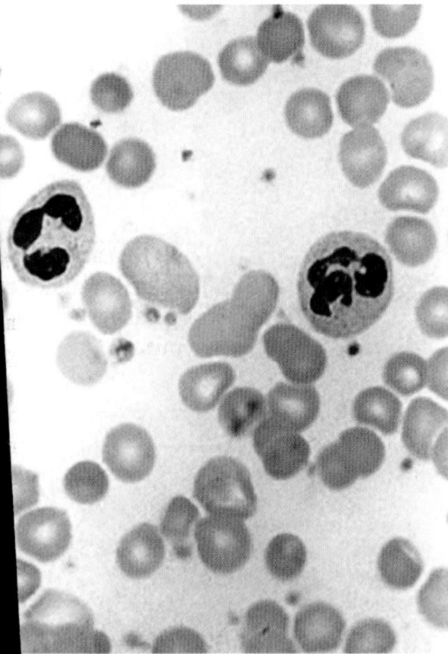

ophil structure.

es

and structure

gs 4.5 and 4.6) tend to be the largest od cell, measuring up to 25 μm in diam- a large, kidney-shaped nucleus. Nucleoli nt, giving the nucleus a 'moth-eaten' e cytoplasm contains many lysosomes ke spaces producing a 'ground-glass' crotubules, microfilaments, pinocytotic vesicles and filo- or pseudopodia are present around the edge of the cell.

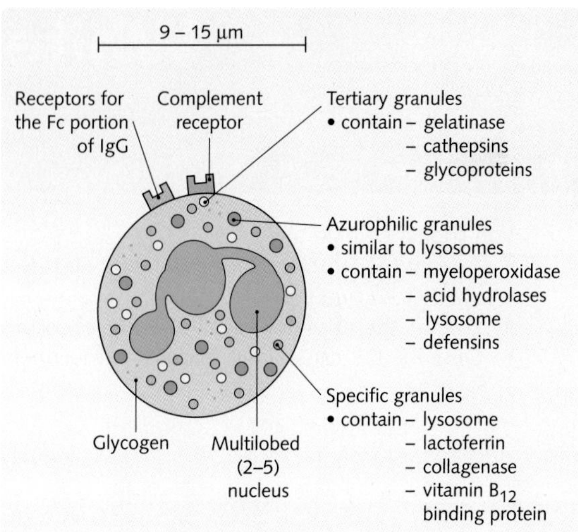

Fig. 4.4 Normal neutrophils have a characteristic multilobed nucleus (connected by chromatin). The cytoplasm is granular.

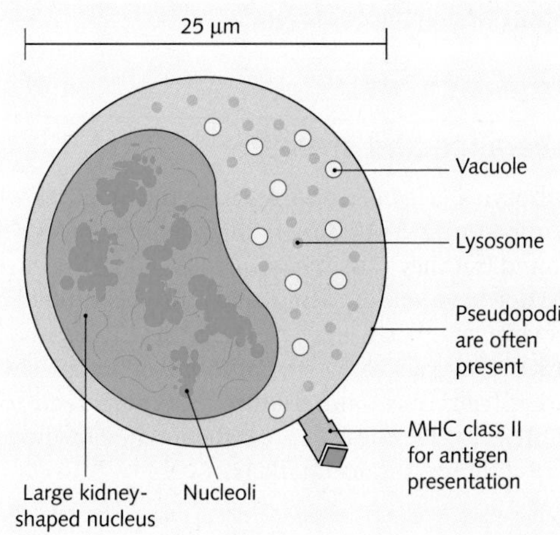

Fig. 4.5 Monocyte structure. MHC, major histocompatibility complex.

Location

Monocytes spend only a few days in the blood before migrating into the tissues, where they differentiate to become macrophages. Macrophages survive for several months to years in connective tissue.

Function

Monocytes form the reticuloendothelial system, which is primarily involved in phagocytosis. They destroy dead or defunct cells and ingest foreign material. Antigens are processed and can be presented to lymphocytes to initiate an adaptive immune response. Macrophages also have a pro-inflammatory function, releasing a variety of cytokines.

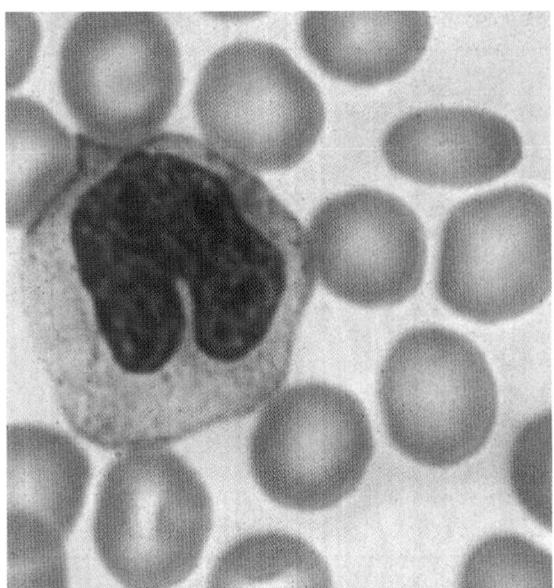

Fig. 4.6 Normal monocytes are large. The nucleus tends to be folded, not lobed, and the cytoplasm contains very fine granules.

Eosinophils

Appearance and structure

Eosinophils (Figs 4.7 and 4.8) are similar to neutrophils but are larger and measure 12–17 μm in diameter. Their nucleus is sausage-shaped and usually bilobed. They have a small, central Golgi apparatus and limited rough endoplasmic reticulum and mitochondria. Eosinophils contain large, ovoid, specific granules and azurophilic granules. The specific granules (1–1.5 μm long) have a crystalloid centre containing major basic protein, eosinophilic cationic protein and eosinophil-derived neurotoxin. The outside of the granule contains several enzymes, including histaminase, peroxidase and cathepsin.

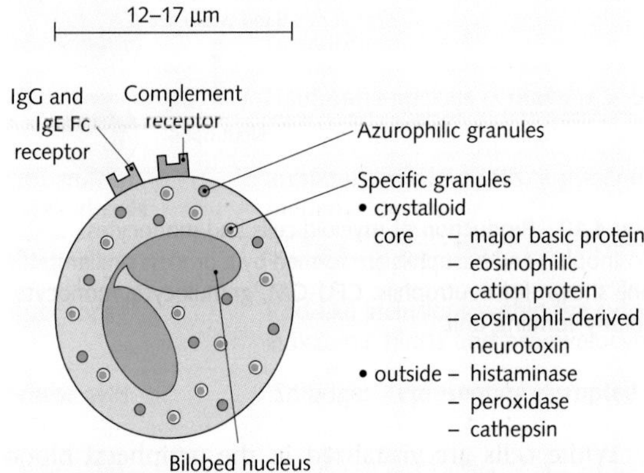

Fig. 4.7 Eosinophil structure.

Location

They are primarily found in the tissues, spending less than 1 hour in blood.

Function

Their primary function is to combat parasitic infection. Eosinophils are seen in allergic and certain malignant disease processes. They also phagocytose antigen–antibody complexes.

Basophils

Appearance and structure

Basophils (Figs 4.8 and 4.9) are 14–16 μm in diameter with a bilobed, 'S-shaped' nucleus. They are named after their highly basophilic cytoplasmic specific granules, but also contain azurophilic granules. Specific granules (0.5 μm in diameter) are large, membrane-bound, round or oval structures. They push into the plasma membrane causing a 'roughened perimeter'. The granules contain heparin, histamine, chemotactic factors and peroxidase.

Location

Basophils undergo maturation in the bone marrow over 2–7 days. They are found in the peripheral blood, and last for up to 2 weeks.

Function

Basophils are functionally very similar to mast cells, although they are of two different lineages. Unlike basophils, mast cells are located in the tissues. Through interactions with immunoglobulin E (IgE) basophils cause local inflammatory responses. Basophils are not very well understood and the extent to which they participate in immune reactions in vivo is unclear. They are thought to mediate immediate (type I) hypersensitivity reactions such as asthma and anaphylaxis (see Chapter 12), along with mast cells. Recent studies in mice show that basophils are important in a new pathway of anaphylaxis involving IgG and platelet-activating factor (PAF).

DIFFERENTIATION OF WHITE CELLS

Granulocytes and monocytes are formed in the bone marrow from a common precursor cell (CFU-GM). Their differentiation pathways are shown in Figure 4.10.

Neutrophils usually develop within bone marrow, but with increased demand, e.g. severe infection, band cells may be seen in blood. Using a neutrophil with a three-lobed nucleus as a marker for normal granulocyte maturation, a shift of development to either the right or left can be seen. Left shift is indicated by the presence of immature

REACTIVE PROLIFERATION OF WHITE CELLS

Leucocytosis

Leucocytosis is an increase in the total white cell count ($>11 \times 10^9$/L). One leucocyte type, most commonly neutrophils, tends to predominate, with small increases in other types. Diseases associated with increases in white-cell count are listed in Figure 4.14.

HINTS AND TIPS

A general increase in white blood cells is called a leucocytosis and in lymphocytes is called a lymphocytosis; a specific increase in granulocyte counts is known as a granulocytosis. If neutrophils, eosinophils or basophils are selectively raised, then the terms neutrophilia, eosinophilia or basophilia are used, respectively.

LEUCOPENIA

- Leucopenia: reduction in white blood cells ($<4 \times 10^9$/L), most commonly neutrophils
- Neutropenia (granulocytopenia): reduction in neutrophils ($<1.8 \times 10^9$/L)
- Agranulocytosis: severe, acute reduction in neutrophils ($<0.5 \times 10^9$/L in peripheral blood). Is associated with risk of infection and can be fatal
- Lymphopenia: reduction in lymphocyte count ($<1.5 \times 10^9$/L).

Causes of neutropenia and agranulocytosis

- Inadequate granulopoiesis
- Accelerated removal of granulocytes
- Drug-induced neutropenia.

Inadequate granulopoiesis

Reduced or ineffective production of neutrophils in the bone marrow results in neutropenia. This can be generalized bone marrow failure such as:

- Aplastic anaemia (see p. 34): a group of disorders characterized by anaemia, thrombocytopenia and neutropenia

Fig. 4.14 Diseases associated with increased white-cell counts

Cell type	Associated diseases	Examples
Leucocytes	Infection, inflammation, allergy and malignancy	
Neutrophils	Bacterial infections Acute inflammation or tissue necrosis Neoplasms Myeloproliferative disorders Metabolic disorders	Pyogenic bacteria Infarction, surgery, burns, myositis, vasculitis Carcinoma, lymphoma, melanoma Chronic myeloid leukaemia, myelofibrosis Eclampsia, gout, diabetic ketoacidosis
Eosinophils	Parasitic infestation Allergic reaction Skin disease Neoplasms Infections	Malaria, hookworm, filariasis, schistosomiasis Asthma, hay fever Pemphigus, eczema, psoriasis, dermatitis herpetiformis, urticaria Hodgkin's disease, metabolic carcinoma, chronic myeloid leukaemia Convalescent phase of any infection
Basophils	Myeloproliferative disorders	Chronic myeloid leukaemia, polycythaemia rubra vera
Lymphocytes	Acute infections Chronic infections Neoplasms	Infectious mononucleosis, pertussis, rubella, viral infection TB, syphilis Chronic lymphocytic leukaemia, lymphoma
Monocytes	Chronic infections and inflammatory diseases Neoplasms	TB, bacterial endocarditis, protozoa Lymphomas, myelodysplastic syndromes

TB, tuberculosis.

- Invasion of the bone marrow in leukaemias and lymphomas. Neutropenia is accompanied by anaemia and thrombocytopenia
- Megaloblastic anaemia due to vitamin B_{12} or folate deficiency (see p. 25): this leads to impaired DNA synthesis, resulting in abnormal granulocyte precursors that are more susceptible to destruction.
- Chemotherapy
- Myelodysplasia.

Or a specific failure of neutrophil production:

- Congenital (Kostmann's syndrome)
- Exposure to certain drugs (Fig. 4.15)
- Cyclical.

Accelerated removal of granulocytes

- Immune-mediated destruction:
  - Idiopathic
  - Secondary to other autoimmune diseases, e.g. Felty's syndrome (rheumatoid arthritis associated with leucopenia and splenomegaly)
  - Due to drug therapy, e.g. chlorpromazine
  - Hypersensitivity and anaphylaxis
- Hypersplenism causing splenic sequestration of neutrophils
- Severe infection (e.g. typhoid, miliary tuberculosis) resulting in increased peripheral utilization.

Fig. 4.15 Drugs that can cause neutropenia

- Chemotherapy
- Analgesic and anti-inflammatory agents (aminopyrine, phenylbutazone)
- Hypnotics and sedatives (clozapine, mianserin, imipramine)
- Antimalarials (chloroquine)
- Diuretics and antihypertensives (furosemide)
- Anticonvulsants (phenytoin, carbamazepine)
- Antithyroid drugs (carbimazole)
- Antibiotics (chloramphenicol, co-trimoxazole, imipenem)
- Hypoglycaemic agents (tolbutamide)
- Antirheumatoid drugs (gold, sulfasalazine)

Drug-induced neutropenia

Drug-induced neutropenia is increasing in frequency. Two mechanisms operate:

1. Direct toxicity: interference with protein synthesis or cell replication of pluripotent stem cells causes a dose-dependent, generalized bone marrow depression.
2. Immune-mediated destruction of neutrophils: this is not related to drug dose and usually occurs early in the course of the therapy.

Causes of lymphopenia

Lymphopenia is most commonly secondary to minor, community-acquired viral infections. Other causes of lymphopenia are:

- Corticosteroid and other immunosuppressive therapy
- Trauma or surgery
- Cushing's syndrome
- Systemic lupus erythematosus (SLE)
- Hodgkin's lymphoma
- HIV infection and AIDS.

Mild lymphopenia has little in the way of clinical consequences and it is only in situations of prolonged severe lymphopenia, such as that seen in HIV-positive patients, where significantly clinical sequelae are evident.

Haema ... cies 5

Objectives

You should be a

- Understand t ... blood cells
- Compare the
- Outline the a
- Explain the d

INTRODUCTION TO HAEMATOLOGICAL MALIGNANCIES

Haematological malignancies may affect the bone marrow, lymph nodes and blood. Like other malignancies, they begin with the formation of an aberrant cell due to somatic (genetic) mutation. These mutations occur as a result of genetic and environmental factors which are often specific to the tumour involved and result in increased proliferation, reduced apoptosis and reduced differentiation. All subsequent proliferating cells are identical (clones) to the original aberrant cell. A neoplastic clone can arise at any stage in development, from the myeloid stem cell and in either one of the three lineages, or from a lymphoid clone.

Haematological malignancies are complicated and are classified differently by different individuals and organizations. They are broken down into separate categories according to the current perception of the cell of origin, the tissue in which they usually arise, the molecular basis of the clonal proliferation and any specific characteristics. We have attempted to classify them as simply as possible:

- Myeloproliferative disorders—bone marrow disorders resulting in excess of one or more type of myeloid cell (i.e. a proliferation of blood cells)
- Myelodysplastic syndromes—diverse group of bone marrow disorders that result in the clonal production of abnormal (dysplastic) myeloid cells. These cells fail to mature properly, resulting in blast (immature) cells
- Leukaemias—a collection of diseases that result in a clonal proliferation of white blood cells
- Lymphomas—clonal proliferations of lymphoid cells, mainly from lymph nodes and extranodal tissue
- Myeloma—malignant proliferation of plasma cells.

Managing haematological malignancies is difficult and is almost always performed by specialists. Often chemotherapeutic drugs and immunosuppressants are used. More targeted treatments have emerged because of developments in molecular and cell biology, as well as cytogenetics. Examples of newer therapies include:

- Monoclonal anti-B cell antibodies (rituximab)
- Anti-angiogenic therapy (thalidomide and lenalidomide)
- Purine analogues (fludarabine)
- Proteosome inhibitors (bortezomib)
- ATRA (all trans-retinoic acid) targets the cytogenetic translocation in acute promyelocytic leukaemia
- Specific treatment to target the mutation of acute myeloid leukaemia (imatinib).

This does not mean that more standard therapies have been abandoned, but that newer treatments are improving the remission rates and the time to relapse in many haematological malignancies.

We discuss some important haematological investigations at the end of this chapter.

Myeloproliferative neoplasms

These disorders arise as a result of the neoplastic clonal proliferation of multipotent myeloid stem cells, which are capable of following one or more differentiation pathways (Fig. 5.1).

Myeloproliferative disorders encompass:

- Primary polycythaemia (polycythaemia rubra vera)
- Myelofibrosis
- Primary thrombocythaemia (essential thrombocythaemia)
- Chronic myeloid leukaemia—this disorder is discussed later. See p. 49.

Myeloproliferative disorders are not malignant neoplasms but can sometimes evolve into acute myeloid leukaemia.

Fig. 5.1 Possible differentiation pathways of multipotent myeloid stem cells and associated myeloproliferative disorders.

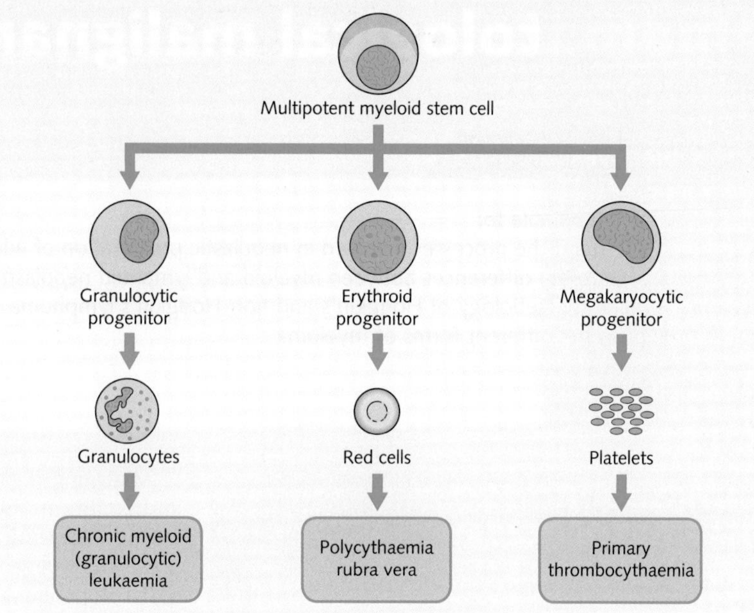

Primary thrombocythaemia (essential thrombocythaemia)

This is a disorder involving clonal proliferation of the megakaryocyte cell line, although it is, in reality, a stem cell disorder. A sustained raised platelet count ($> 450 \times 10^9$/L) is the dominant feature. It usually presents after the age of 50 but can occur at any age. About half of affected individuals are asymptomatic at diagnosis, thus it is often an incidental finding on a routine blood test.

The disorder is characterized clinically by thrombosis or bleeding. Haemorrhage is more common with higher platelet counts, e.g. $> 1000 \times 10^9$/L. Some patients develop acquired von Willebrand's disease because the high level of platelets affects the von Willebrand protein (see p. 66). There are raised levels of abnormal megakaryocytes in the bone marrow. Splenic atrophy, as a result of microinfarcts, may occur but is rarely clinically relevant.

Treatment involves the reduction of platelet levels by hydroxycarbamide, α-interferon or anagrelide (second-line therapy). Aspirin is commonly used to reduce thrombotic risk.

Primary polycythaemia (polycythaemia rubra vera)

A proliferative abnormality of stem cells gives rise to increased numbers of red cells, often with an increase in the numbers of neutrophils and platelets. The red-cell precursors are inappropriately sensitive to insulin-like growth factor +/− interleukin-3 and therefore do not require erythropoietin (EPO) to avoid apoptosis. The majority of patients with primary polycythaemia have a gain-of-function mutation of the Janus kinase (JAK) 2 gene. This mutation is also present in a high proportion of patients with primary thrombocythaemia and idiopathic myelofibrosis.

Polycythaemia rubra vera presents insidiously after the age of 40, with symptoms attributable to hyperviscosity and vascular occlusion. These symptoms include headache, dizziness and stroke. Thrombosis is the most common serious complication. Clinical signs include plethora, splenomegaly and hepatomegaly.

Haematological findings include:

- Raised packed cell volume, red-cell mass, haemoglobin and red-cell count
- Raised white-cell count (neutrophils)
- Raised neutrophil alkaline phosphatase
- Raised platelet count
- Hyperplasia of erythroid, granulocytic and megakaryocytic cells in bone marrow
- Decreased serum EPO
- Increased plasma urate.

Treatment is by venesection reducing the packed cell volume to within normal limits. Aspirin offers a slight reduction in thrombotic risk. Other therapies, reserved for patients with higher thrombotic risk, include cytotoxic drugs (hydroxycarbamide is the drug of choice) and irradiation of the bone marrow using ^{32}P. However, ^{32}P can cause more malignant transformation. Some patients develop acute leukaemia or myelofibrosis. The main causes of death are thromboses and acute leukaemia. However, if the red cell count is kept low, the prognosis is good. Modern therapy extends 50% survival beyond 10 years compared to historical figures of less than 2 years.

Myelofibrosis

Also known as primary myelosclerosis, idiopathic myelofibrosis is characterized by clonal proliferation of pluripotent stem cells. Idiopathic myelofibrosis can be preceded by other myeloproliferative conditions; 25% of cases are preceded by polycythaemia rubra vera. Bone marrow is replaced by fibrous tissue produced by fibroblasts in conjunction with proliferation of dysplastic megakaryocytes. Extramedullary metaplasia is also a feature, with the spleen being the primary site, resulting in massive splenomegaly. The same process may also result in hepatomegaly. The disease affects individuals from middle-age onwards. Clinical features include constitutional symptoms of weight loss, night sweats and fever, or those relating to anaemia (fatigue, shortness of breath and palpitations) or splenomegaly (abdominal pain due to the mass effect). Laboratory features at presentation include anaemia, leucocytosis and thrombocytosis. The blood film is often diagnostic, revealing:

- Granulocyte precursor cells
- Nucleated red blood cell precursors
- Tear-drop poikilocytosis (tear-drop-shaped erythrocytes).

Supportive care (including transfusions of red cells and platelets) can be useful, and splenectomy or splenic irradiation is sometimes beneficial. Chemotherapy with hydroxycarbamide or α-interferon 2b can slow or reverse fibrosis. Median survival is 5 years. Approximately 10% of cases transform into acute myeloblastic leukaemia (AML).

Myelodysplastic syndromes

Myelodysplasias are acquired neoplastic disorders of bone marrow, with replacement of normal cells by a clone of abnormal (dysplastic) cells. These cells are unable to mature normally, usually affecting at least two cell lines (erythrocytes, granulocytes, monocytes or platelets) and as a result blast cells may accumulate. The dysmorphic cells are easily recognizable on microscopy with an increasing blast cell count indicating a poorer prognosis. Common features of myelodysplasias include the following:

- Occurs most commonly in the elderly and in males
- Slowly progressive disease, often with anaemia, easy bruising or bleeding and infections
- May follow chemo- and/or radiotherapy for another condition
- Normal or increased bone marrow cellularity
- Cytopenias
- Progression to AML.

The traditional classification was the French-American-British (FAB) classification, but this was revised by the World Health Organization (WHO) in 2008 (Fig. 5.2). Prognosis is calculated using the International Prognostic Scoring System (IPSS) based on the percentage of bone marrow blast cells. Generally speaking, the greater number of blasts and the presence of cytopenias indicate a worse prognosis.

Fig. 5.2 The French-American-British (FAB) and World Health Organization (WHO) classifications of myelodysplastic syndrome subtypes

FAB classification	WHO classification
Refractory anaemia (RA) – bone marrow blasts < 5%, < 1% blasts in the blood	RA Refractory cytopenia and multilineage dysplasia (RCMD) Myelodysplastic syndrome with isolated deletion of chromosome 5q Myelodysplastic syndrome – unclassified
Refractory anaemia with ringed sideroblasts (RARS) – as for RA with ringed sideroblasts > 15% of erythroblasts	RARS Refractory cytopenias with multilineage dysplasia and ringed sideroblasts
RA with excess blasts (RAEB) – bone marrow blasts 5–20%, blasts in the blood < 5%	RAEB-1 (5–9% bone marrow blasts) RAEB-2 (10–19% bone marrow blasts)
RAEB in transformation (RAEBt) – as RAEB but bone marrow blasts 20–30% or Auer rods present	Patients with > 20% blasts are now recognized as having acute myeloid leukaemia
Chronic myelomonocytic leukaemia (CMML) – any of the above + > 1.0×10^9/L monocytes	Now removed from myelodysplastic syndromes and part of the myelodysplastic-myeloproliferative overlap syndromes.

As well as the morphological appearance, cytogenetic changes will influence prognosis and treatment. Thus cytogenetic analysis should be undertaken at presentation. Treatment, until recently, has been mainly supportive with blood and platelet transfusions, as well as antibiotics if needed. There is evidence that the use of biological therapy such as EPO and G-CSF will improve survival in some patients. Younger patients with more advanced disease will be treated with intensive chemotherapy and possibly bone marrow transplantation. There may also be a role for thalidomide and its derivatives.

Leukaemia

Features common to leukaemias

Leukaemias are a group of disorders characterized by accumulation of clonal white blood cells in bone marrow. The leukaemic 'blast' cells are non-functional and replace normal bone marrow, encroaching on normal haemopoietic cell development. This leads to anaemia, neutropenia and thrombocytopenia.

HINTS AND TIPS

Many symptoms of leukaemia are due to organ infiltration by leukaemic cells. Organs that are commonly involved include:

- Bones
- Lymph nodes
- Liver and spleen
- Skin
- Central nervous system.

Classification of leukaemia is based on:

- Cell lineage (lymphoid or myeloid)
- Developmental stage of leukaemic cells: acute leukaemia involves proliferation of immature cells (blasts) and, untreated, is usually rapidly fatal; chronic leukaemia involves more mature cells, and a more prolonged course is characteristic.

Acute leukaemias are myeloblastic (AML) or lymphoblastic (ALL).

The management of patients with leukaemia is done by haematologists in the hospital setting.

Acute myeloid leukaemia

AML (sometimes called acute myeloblastic leukaemia) is the most common leukaemia found in adults, although it can occur at any age. It is a clonal disorder of myeloid origin, producing primitive blast cells that invade bone marrow, suppressing all normal cell lines. These blast cells can be seen on peripheral blood films. The majority of cases have no known cause, although they can progress from both the myeloproliferative and myelodysplastic disorders. The incidence increases with age (median 70 years) with an average of 4 per 100,000 per year. The 5-year survival rate is over 50% in children and about 30–50% in adults who are treated. Elderly patients have a poorer prognosis. AML is associated with:

- Radiation exposure
- Toxins: benzene, alkylating agents
- Hereditary abnormalities, e.g. Down syndrome
- Pre-existing haematological disease: chronic myeloid leukaemia (CML), myelodysplastic syndromes.

Usually, however, there is no obvious cause.

Patients are often acutely unwell at presentation and can present with:

- Anaemia, malaise, sweats, weight loss
- Infections (chest, mouth, skin)
- Bleeding
- Skin infiltration (gums M4/5)
- Leucostasis.

HINTS AND TIPS

Leucostatic symptoms occur when excess white blood cells increase the viscosity of the blood. This causes occlusions in the heart, lungs and brain. Symptoms include reduced consciousness, retinal haemorrhages and pulmonary infiltrates.

AML also has both a FAB and a WHO classification. The FAB classification divides AML into eight subtypes based on morphology and cytochemistry M0–M7. The WHO classification includes more recently identified molecular abnormalities which have prognostic significance. Chromosome rearrangements have prognostic value with t(15;17), t(8;21) and inversion of 16 having better outcomes than monosomy 7. t(15;17) is the specific mutation associated with acute promyelocytic leukaemia. It is the only form of AML which responds to all trans-retinoic acid (ATRA)

Like other leukaemias, AML is treated by specialists and often as part of a clinical trial. It is treated in two phases:

- Induction—to achieve remission
- Consolidation (intensification).

To achieve remission anthracycline-based chemotherapy regimens are used. Provided patients remain in remission at the end of consolidation, autologous or allogenic stem cell transplantation is then an option for some patients. Survival is best in younger patients.

The haematological consequences of AML are treated to improve symptoms and outcome. This includes transfusions of red cells/platelets, leukopheresis to reduce blood viscosity and the prevention/treatment of infection.

AML

Patients usually present with a short history of recurrent sore throats or easy bruising. A blood count reveals anaemia and thrombocytopenia. The white-cell blood count (WBC) may be low or high but there will be blast cells in the bone marrow which may also be seen in the blood. These patients require immediate admission to hospital. If they are not treated with intensive chemotherapy they will rapidly die of sepsis or bleeding.

Stem cell transplantation (SCT) involves using high-dose chemotherapy (and or radiotherapy) to destroy all cancerous cells in the bone marrow, and they are then replaced with (disease-free) haemopoietic stem cells. The new stem cells can be sourced from the bone marrow, hence the name bone marrow transplant, or can be a peripheral blood stem cell transplant (PBSCT).

These cells can come from the patient's own body (autologous SCT) or from another person (allogenic SCT). This other person is usually a human leucocyte antigen (HLA)-matched relative, in order to prevent host immune rejection, which is known as graft-versus-host disease (GVHD). Immunosuppressive drugs such as cyclosporin and methotrexate are used to reduce the incidence of GVHD.

Other complications of SCT include graft failure, opportunistic infections, and interstitial pneumonitis.

HINTS AND TIPS

The term 'remission' refers to the disappearance of the signs and symptoms of the disease. This can be permanent or a patient may suffer from a relapse. Sometimes 'complete remission' is used to describe a clinical disappearance as well as a biochemical or histological return to normality.

Chronic myeloid leukaemia

CML, also known as chronic granulocytic leukaemia, is a progressive accumulation of mature myeloid cells in blood and bone marrow. At presentation the white-cell count is usually in the range 20–200 x 10^9/L (normal range 4–11 $\times$ 10^9/L), but can be much higher. These are mainly myelocytes and neutrophils but blasts are detectable in the early, chronic phase. An increase in basophils is characteristic. It accounts for 15% of all leukaemias. The average incidence is 1 in 100,000, peaking between 40 and 60 years of age. It is rare in children and there is a slight male preponderance. Clinically, it runs a predictable course, with three identifiable phases of the disease:

1. Chronic
2. Accelerated
3. Blast crisis (AML/ALL).

People normally present in the chronic phase following an incidental finding on a full blood count or with constitutional (malaise, weight loss, sweats) or leucostatic symptoms. Many patients will quickly transform to an accelerated or blast crisis stage, if untreated.

The Philadelphia chromosome is a pathognomonic translocation between chromosomes 9 and 22, written as t(9:22), associated with CML. This translocation, found in granulocytic, erythrocytic and megakaryocytic precursor cells, fuses parts of two genes (BCR–ABL) to create an abnormal tyrosine kinase, which plays a pivotal role in the genesis of chronic phase CML. Tyrosine kinase inhibitors (TKI) are now the cornerstone of CML treatment, as opposed to chemotherapeutic agents, which were popular in the past. A TKI, imatinib (traded as Glivec), is now first line for the chronic phase of CML, and provides good remission rates. Bone marrow transplantation is potentially curative, especially in young patients; however, the benefits of treatment must be weighed against the risks of transplantation.

Median survival before the introduction of imatinib was 5½ years. Short term (at 5 years) observational studies show that imatinib produces better complete cytogenetic remission than other therapies, but long-term (> 10 years) studies are ongoing. 65% of patients started on imatinib remain well at 10 years. Good prognostic factors include:

- Youth
- Small spleen at presentation
- Low white-cell count at presentation.

Acute lymphoblastic leukaemia

ALL accounts for 80% of all childhood leukaemias and 60% of cases present before 20 years of age. It is the most common cancer in children. The peak incidence occurs between 2 and 10 years of age. Presentation outside of this range confers a poorer prognosis. The most common presenting symptoms are fatigue, bruising, bleeding, infections and hepatosplenomegaly. ALL may be associated with:

- Radiation
- Chemicals
- Down syndrome.

However, usually there is no obvious cause.

In 80% of cases, the blast cells are of B cell origin. ALL is more responsive to combination chemotherapy than AML and long-term remission rates of around 80% in children are attained. The overall survival rate in adults is 35%. Cure rates are highest in girls over 2 and under 10 years of age. The Philadelphia chromosome is seen in 10–20% of cases and is associated with a poor outcome.

Chronic lymphocytic leukaemia

CLL occurs most frequently in people over the age of 60 years (median age 65) and accounts for 25% of all leukaemias. It is twice as common in men as in women, with a total incidence of 3–4 per 10,000. CLL arises from a proliferation of neoplastic lymphoid cells (B cells), which infiltrate the marrow, lymph nodes, spleen and liver. It is a slowly progressing, low-grade disorder. Patients commonly present with painless lymphadenopathy and anaemia. Because of diminished immunity they may present with a chest infection. On a blood film, leukaemic cells resemble mature lymphocytes, although typical 'smear cells' are also seen. The combination of a typical peripheral blood film and characteristic immunophenotype of the leukaemic cells is enough to make the diagnosis. Disease transformation into prolymphocytic leukaemia occurs rarely and usually after several years. Median survival is 5–8 years and treatment (chemotherapy or stem cell transplantation) is usually aimed at limiting rather than curing the disease. The introduction of combination chemotherapy which includes rituximab has improved the remission rate. Many elderly patients will die of an unrelated condition because of the slowly progressive nature of the disease.

Malignant lymphomas

Lymphomas are a group of neoplastic disorders characterized by the proliferation of a primitive cell which produces clonal expansion of lymphoid cells. They primarily involve the lymph nodes and extranodal lymphoid tissue, e.g. mucosal-associated lymphoid tissue (MALT) and spleen. Malignant lymphomas are divided into two categories:

1. Non-Hodgkin's lymphoma
2. Hodgkin's disease (Hodgkin's lymphoma).

HINTS AND TIPS

Although it is easy to think of leukaemias as disease of the bone marrow and lymphomas as disease of the lymph nodes, remember that leukaemic cells are found in the blood and that lymphoma cells commonly spread to the bone marrow and blood.

Hodgkin's disease

Hodgkin's disease (HD) characteristically affects young people in the third and fourth decades of life and is more common in men. Environmental factors associated with increased risk of HD include Epstein-Barr virus (EBV) and immunosuppression.

Diagnosis requires a lymph node biopsy showing the presence of pathognomonic Reed–Sternberg (RS) cells or derivatives, typically mixed with a variable inflammatory infiltrate. Disease severity is directly proportional to the number of RS cells found in the lesions and indirectly linked to the number of lymphocytes in the lesions. The RS cells are neoplastic derivatives of B cells with a dysfunctional immunoglobulin gene. RS cells are bi- or multinucleated, with prominent eosinophilic nucleoli, giving an 'owl's-eye' appearance.

The clinical features of HD are shown in Figure 5.3.

Ninety-five per cent of HD is termed classical HD, as opposed to nodular lymphocyte-predominant Hodgkin's lymphoma (NLPHL). Classical HD has been classified into four histological subtypes:

- Nodular sclerosing—most common subtype of HD. Unlike other types it is more common in women. Collagen bands divide lymph nodes into nodules
- Lymphocyte-rich—larger number of lymphocytes, conferring a better prognosis
- Mixed cellularity—fewer lymphocytes and more RS cells than lymphocyte-rich form
- Lymphocyte-depleted—RS cells are present in large number, with relatively few lymphocytes. This subtype has the poorest prognosis of all subtypes of HD.

Although histological composition is an important prognostic factor, clinical staging (Ann Arbor staging) is the most accurate indicator of long-term prognosis in HD (Fig. 5.4).

Treatment depends on stage. Many patients require treatment with both combination chemotherapy and radiotherapy. Although this results in remission for many there are risks (Fig. 5.5). Modern treatment aims to try and reduce dual therapy as much as possible but

Fig. 5.3 Clinical features of Hodgkin's disease

- Painless, non-tender lymphadenopathy: cervical then axillary nodes are most common, mediastinal in 10%
- Splenomegaly (rarely massive)
- Respiratory symptoms (mediastinal mass → superior vena cava obstruction)
- Pruritus
- Constitutional symptoms
  - weight loss
  - sweats (often more severe at night)
  - high swinging 'Pel-Ebstein' fever
  - alcohol-induced lymph node pain

Fig. 5.4 Ann Arbor staging of malignant lymphomas (mainly used for HD)

Stage	Sites of involvement
I	Disease limited to single region of nodes or one extranodal site
II	Disease at two sites on the same side of the diaphragm
III	Disease at several sites on both sides of the diaphragm (includes spleen)
IV	Spread of disease to extralymphatic structures, e.g. bone marrow, gut, lung, liver

A: no symptoms
B: weight loss, sweats, fever

Fig. 5.5 Complications of chemotherapy and radiotherapy in Hodgkin's Disease

Chemotherapy	Radiotherapy
AML	AML
Male and female infertility	Secondary solid tumours especially colon, thyroid, lung, breast and bone
Tumour lysis syndrome	Hypothyroidism
	Cardiovascular disease

some patients will continue to require this. In addition, patients with all lymphomas should receive the polyvalent pneumococcal and influenza vaccines.

Both chemotherapy and radiotherapy are associated serious complications, some of which are shown in Figure 5.5.

Tumour lysis syndrome (TLS)

This is a serious metabolic complication of chemotherapy in cancers treatment, especially in relation to acute leukaemias and poorly differentiated lymphomas. As the cancerous cells are destroyed they release their intracellular components into the circulation resulting in hyperkalaemia, hyperuricaemia and hyperphosphataemia. High levels of phosphate bind to plasma calcium resulting in hypocalcaemia. These electrolyte abnormalities can result in renal failure, arrhythmias and sudden death. High urate levels can precipitate acute attacks of gout. In order to prevent TLS all patients should receive allopurinol (a xanthine oxidase inhibitor, which reduces production of urate), in addition to IV hydration.

Non-Hodgkin's lymphomas

Non-Hodgkin's lymphomas (NHL) are a group of malignant diseases involving lymphoid cells, and five times more common than HD. Around 85% of NHL are of B-cell origin. Incidence of NHL rises with age and is more common in men than in women. There are several aetiological factors associated with NHL, including:

- Infections, e.g. EBV and human T cell lymphotrophic virus 1
- Immunodeficiency, e.g. immunosuppressive therapy, solid organ or stem cell transplants, HIV
- Autoimmune disorders
- Irradiation and carcinogens
- Inherited disorders, e.g. ataxia telangiectasia.

The incidence of NHL has increased since the 1970s, probably because of increases in the number of immunodeficient people.

NHL tends to have more extranodal involvement than HD. The features of NHL are outlined in Figure 5.6.

Initially, the 30 or so NHLs were classified under the Revised European American Lymphoma (REAL) classification, however this has been superseded by a WHO classification.

Clinically there are two categories of NHL:

- Low-grade: more indolent and less aggressive. Longer median survival (approximately 10 years), but cannot usually be cured
- High-grade: more aggressive and rapidly growing. Chemotherapies can target these rapidly growing cells, thus a significant proportion can be cured.

HINTS AND TIPS

Traditional chemotherapeutic agents prevent cell division and therefore affect all dividing cells. This action is of benefit when used against the rapidly dividing cancer cells, but it also damages normal cells. A new generation of pharmacological agents are aimed specifically at affected cells. A monoclonal antibody against CD20+ve B-cells, known as rituximab, is now used extensively in all cancers of B-cell origin.

Fig. 5.6 Features of non-Hodgkin's lymphoma

- Superficial, asymmetric, painless lymphadenopathy
- Fever, night sweats and weight loss
- Oropharyngeal involvement (5–10%)
- Cytopenias due to marrow failure or autoimmunity
- Abdominal disease (spleen, liver, MALT and retroperitoneal/mesenteric nodes)

MALT, mucosal-associated lymphoid tissue.

Management depends on the specific type of NHL. NHLs tend to be managed, much like HD, using chemotherapy with or without radiotherapy. High-grade NHLs are normally treated more aggressively.

Some specific NHLs include:

High-grade

- Diffuse large B-cell NHL—between one-third and one-half of all NHL. These tend to respond well to treatment. Currently rituximab is recommended, in combination with the CHOP (cyclophosphamide, doxorubicin, vincristine and prednisolone) chemotherapeutic regimen. Together, they are referred to as R-CHOP
- Mantle cell lymphoma—approximately 5% of NHL. Can be very aggressive, with most patients suffering from advanced disease by the time they present. Often responds to the R-CHOP regime
- Burkitt's lymphoma—this highly aggressive B-cell NHL mostly affects children, and is prevalent in Central Africa. There is a strong association with EBV. Interestingly, the endemic form of Burkitt's lymphoma commonly affects the jaw, as well as abdominal organs. Treatment is with combination chemotherapy and rituximab.

Low-grade

- Follicular lymphoma—accounts for approximately one-quarter of all NHL, and is the most common low-grade NHL. Stages I–II disease can be managed with radiotherapy. Stages III–IV require treatment with rituximab and combination chemotherapy.

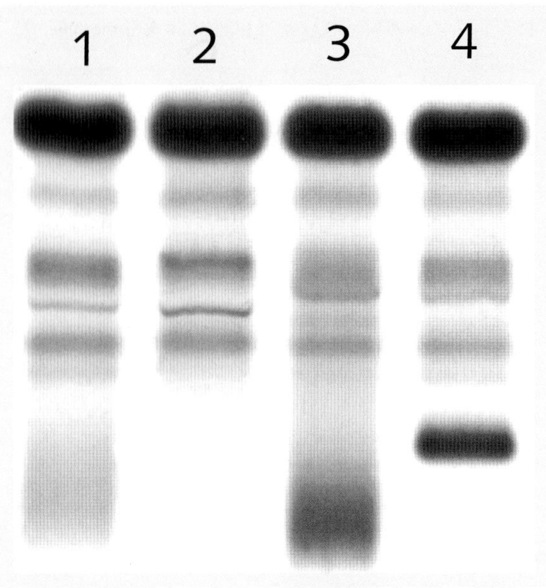

Fig. 5.7 Serum electrophoresis. Electrophoresis uses an electric field to separate proteins or nucleic acids on the basis of size, electric charge and other physical properties. An electric current is passed across a support matrix (e.g. cellulose acetate, polyacrylamide gel) or a solution. As particles travel at different rates (because of their different electrical charge and size), they gradually separate to form bands, which can be visualized by staining. Lane 1, normal sample; lane 2, patient with antibody deficiency; lane 3, patient with infection and polyclonal raised immunoglobulins; lane 4, patient with myeloma and monoclonal immunoglobulin.

Myeloma

Multiple myeloma

Multiple myeloma is a malignant proliferation of plasma cells in bone marrow, which produce a monoclonal paraprotein and/or light chain. The monoclonal immunoglobulin is found in serum, whereas the light chain or Bence Jones protein is found in urine. These monoclonal proteins form a discrete band on the electrophoretic strip (Fig. 5.7). IgG is the most common type of myeloma.

The incidence of multiple myeloma is 4–6/100,000 a year. It is a disease of late middle age and the elderly. The aetiology is unknown, apart from an increased incidence related to exposure to ionizing radiation. The International Staging System (ISS) categorizes myeloma into Stage I, II and III, according to age, laboratory and cytogenetic results.

Clinical features

- Bone destruction such as diffuse osteoporosis and pathological fractures are a common feature. These are described as lytic lesions. They are thought to arise as a result of bone resorption induced by the production of osteoclast-activating factor (OAF) by the myeloma cells. The axial skeleton is most commonly affected (see Fig. 5.8 for the radiographic appearance of multiple myeloma)
- Neurological symptoms due to the compression of the spinal cord or roots by collapsed vertebrae
- Normochromic normocytic anaemia results from marrow infiltration
- Rouleaux formation is seen on blood film due to excess high-molecular-weight proteins in the serum (see Fig. 5.9)
- Repeated infections can occur due to hypogammaglobulinaemia and neutropenia
- Hypercalcaemia occurs in 10% of cases. This is due to increased resorption of bone and is indicative of advanced disease
- Chronic renal failure occurs in 20–30% of patients. Factors that can contribute to renal failure in multiple myeloma are:
  - Increased blood viscosity
  - Hypercalcaemia
  - Renal tubular obstruction by proteinaceous casts
  - Toxic effect of Bence Jones protein on proximal renal tubules
  - Infection

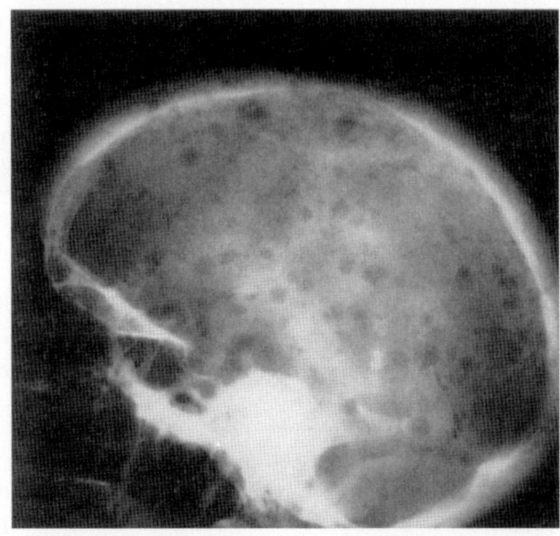

Fig. 5.8 A radiograph of the skull of a patient with multiple myeloma showing many osteolytic bone lesions. Some call this appearance a 'pepper pot skull' (courtesy of Dr M Makris).

  - Dehydration
  - Non-steroidal anti-inflammatory drugs
  - Light-chain deposition in glomeruli
- Amyloidosis (see below) can lead to nephrotic syndrome
- An abnormal bleeding tendency occurs owing to the adverse effect of paraprotein on platelets and coagulation factors.

If myeloma is suspected a bone marrow sample is needed, along with a skeletal survey and both serum protein electrophoresis and immunofixation of urine. A skeletal survey consists of X-rays of the skull, thorax, pelvis and proximal long bones. Diagnosis requires evidence of the following:

- Monoclonal paraprotein in serum and/or urine
- An increased number of (clonal) plasma cells in the bone marrow
- Related organ or tissue damage (including osteolytic bone lesions on skeletal survey).

Complete remission is only possible if a solitary lesion is successfully excised, or a SCT eradicates the diseased cells. Other than this, treatment is not curative. Combination chemotherapy with an alkylating agent, an immune modulator or possibly a proteasome inhibitor is often used. There is a strong role for steroids in first-line treatment. Stem cell transplantation is a possible treatment for a small number of younger patients who respond to first-line treatment. All patients should have their pain addressed adequately, along with sufficient hydration. Patients are routinely given bisphosphonates to inhibit bone resorption.

Solitary myeloma (plasmacytoma)

A plasmacytoma is a solitary tumour found either in the bone or soft tissues, especially the upper respiratory tract. Osseous plasmacytomas usually progress to multiple myeloma. Extraosseous plasmacytomas do not disseminate and, after excision and radiotherapy, prognosis is excellent.

Waldenström's macroglobulinaemia

Waldenström's macroglobulinaemia is a neoplastic monoclonal proliferation of cells derived from the B-cell lineage. It is seen as a low-grade NHL. A monoclonal IgM paraprotein (macroglobulin) is produced, increasing blood viscosity markedly. Tumour cells are found in blood, bone marrow, lymph nodes and spleen. The incidence is 3–6/100,000 a year and is higher in males than in females. Most patients present between the fifth and seventh decade. Survival averages 2–5 years. Bone pain and osteolytic lesions are rare but hyperviscosity syndrome is common but may not always cause

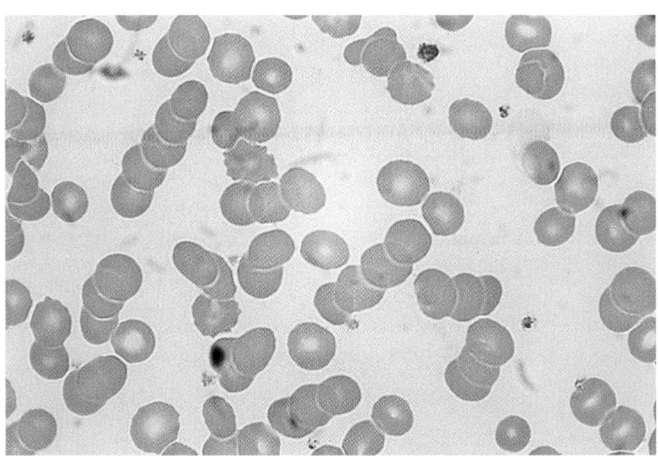

Fig. 5.9 Red cell rouleaux (stacked cells) are seen due to the excess high-molecular-weight proteins in the blood. This is seen in multiple myeloma, as well as inflammatory conditions, connective tissue conditions and diabetes.

symptoms. Where it does, then hyperviscosity syndrome is treated with plasmaphoresis. Macroglobulin interferes with platelet function and coagulation factors, resulting in a tendency to bleed. Management is mainly supportive, but symptomatic patients may require chemotherapy.

Monoclonal gammopathy of undetermined significance

Around 3% of people aged over 65 years have low levels of paraprotein without any symptoms of disease. This condition is termed monoclonal gammopathy of uncertain significance (MGUS). There are < 10% plasma cells in the marrow, no bone lesions, no anaemia and no renal failure; 10% will progress to myeloma within 10 years.

Amyloidosis

Amyloid is a heterogeneous group of proteins that have a fibrillar ultrastructure resulting in the formation of β-pleated sheets. Examples of amyloid proteins include:

- AA: serum amyloid A (SAA), an acute phase protein
- AL: immunoglobulin light chain or fragments.

In amyloidosis, amyloid is deposited in tissues. This can be localized or systemic, with renal impairment being an important problem. Amyloidosis can occur in plasma cell disorders as well as other unrelated disorders, including chronic inflammatory conditions. Treatment may include chemotherapy and is usually done in collaboration with the UK National Amyloidosis Centre.

INVESTIGATIONS OF HAEMATOLOGICAL MALIGNANCIES

Erythrocyte sedimentation rate and plasma viscosity

The erythrocyte sedimentation rate (ESR) is the rate of fall of a column of red cells in plasma over 1 hour. The normal range in men is 1–5 mm/hour and in women it is 5–15 mm/hour. ESR is raised with increased plasma viscosity, which is a more easily automated test. The concentration of proteins (fibrinogen and globulins) in the plasma is the major determinant of viscosity. ESR and plasma viscosity are used as indicators of the acute phase response. ESR is raised in inflammation (including response to infection), malignancy (including myeloma) and anaemia. It is important to remember that a normal increase in ESR occurs with age and during pregnancy.

Bone marrow investigation

Bone marrow smear

Bone marrow smears allow examination of the stages of haemopoiesis. Bone marrow smears are usually stained with Romanowsky dyes, but Perls' Prussian blue may be used to detect iron in macrophages and erythroblasts.

Collection of bone marrow

- Aspiration of bone marrow involves the insertion of a hollow needle into the iliac crest or more rarely the sternum. Individual cell detail can be assessed from aspirates
- Trephine biopsy involves insertion of a large-bore needle into the iliac crest. A core of bone and marrow is obtained, which is examined as a histological specimen. These specimens are useful for assessing marrow architecture and cellularity.

HINTS AND TIPS

Sometimes bone marrow aspiration fails to produce marrow cells, this is known as a 'dry tap'. This is not normally due to poor technique, but is indicative of certain pathologies in the marrow. These include chronic myeloid leukaemia, myelofibrosis and metastatic cancer.

The bone marrow findings in some disorders are listed in Fig. 5.10.

Lymph node biopsy

Lymph nodes are biopsied for histological examination when malignancy is suspected.

Cytogenetic analysis

Cytogenetic analysis is the study of structure and function of chromosomes. Certain cytogenetic abnormalities are strongly associated with specific conditions. Important examples in haematology are:

- t(9;22): this is found mainly in chronic myeloid leukaemia, but also in acute lymphoblastic leukaemia (the altered chromosome 22 is called the Philadelphia chromosome)
- t(14;18): this is associated with follicular lymphoma
- t(8;14): this is associated with Burkitt's lymphoma.

Fig. 5.10 Appearance of the bone marrow in some haematological disorders

Disorder	Bone marrow appearance
Iron-deficiency anaemia	Absent iron stores from macrophages
Megaloblastic anaemia	Hypercellular marrow with megaloblasts present; giant metamyelocytes often seen
Haemolytic anaemia	Hypercellular marrow with erythroid hyperplasia; reduced myeloid/erythroid ratio (usually 2–8)
Aplastic anaemia	Hypocellular marrow
Acute leukaemia	Hypercellular marrow infiltrated with blasts
Chronic lymphocytic leukaemia	Hypercellular marrow with lymphocytic infiltration
Chronic myeloid leukaemia	Hypercellular marrow with granulocytic and megakaryocytic hyperplasia
Multiple myeloma	Increased proportion of plasma cells (often abnormal)
Polycythaemia rubra vera and essential thrombocythaemia	Hypercellular marrow with hyperplasia of all cell lineages
Myelofibrosis	Early—hypercellularity, late—reactive fibrosis of the bone marrow and reduced haemopoiesis

Courtesy of Professor Victor Hoffbrand and Dr John Pettit.

Haemostasis

Objectives

You should be able to:

- Understand the structure and function of platelets, and how they are formed
- Explain different disorders affecting platelets
- Outline the different pathways and substances involved in the coagulation cascade
- Relate the function and disorders of clotting factors
- Discuss different forms of thrombosis and how they arise
- Describe the importance of thromboprophylaxis and methods used to prevent thrombotic disease
- Know how anticoagulants work, including the mechanisms of warfarin and heparin.

Haemostatis is complicated but is based on very simple principles. Humans have evolved a circulatory system that transports vital nutrients around the body at high pressures. If a blood vessel is damaged blood will follow the pressure gradient and leave the vessel, reducing the circulating volume and compromising organ perfusion. We have, therefore, evolved a system, the haemostatic system, which will attempt to arrest any bleeding as quickly as possible.

HINTS AND TIPS

A blood clot located where it was formed is called a thrombus. If it is dislodged and attaches to other vessel it becomes known as a thromboembolism. The presence or formation of a thrombus is referred to as thrombosis.

Three local mechanisms are employed to try to avoid blood loss:

1. Local neurohumoral factors, such as endothelin released by cells adjacent to the injury, induce transient vasoconstriction. Reducing the flow of blood minimizes blood loss as well as maximizing interactions between platelets, clotting factors and the vessel wall.
2. Primary haemostasis utilizes circulating platelets to form an adhesive plug to slow bleeding.
3. Secondary haemostasis (the coagulation cascade) involves circulating plasma proteins. They produce a fibrin network that stabilizes the platelets and traps both red and white blood cells. This stable plug remains until cellular processes repair the damage.

HINTS AND TIPS

Haemostatic response: the arrest of bleeding, involving the physiological processes of the contraction of damaged blood vessels, platelet activation and adhesion, and coagulation.

PLATELETS AND BLOOD COAGULATION

Platelets are disc-shaped, non-nucleated, granule-containing cell fragments with a mean diameter of 2–3 μm (Fig. 6.1). They are formed in the bone marrow from megakaryocyte cytoplasm. The normal lifespan of platelets is 7–10 days and at any time up to one-third are sequestered in the spleen.

Platelet structure and production

The normal discoid circulating shape is maintained by a band of 10–15 parallel microtubules located around the circumference. Platelets have two tubular systems: the dense tubular system and the surface-opening canalicular system. Platelets contain two types of granule, α and δ, which contain molecules involved in platelet aggregation.

Haemopoietic stem cells differentiate to form megakaryoblasts. Megakaryoblasts mature by endomitosis, expanding cytoplasmic volume and increasing the number of nuclear lobes without dividing. This forms a polyploid megakaryocyte, which can produce 2000–7000 platelets. Cytoplasmic processes protrude into sinusoids where they fragment into proplatelets, which then disperse as individual platelets, with the megakaryocyte

Antithrombin deficiency

AT deficiency is an autosomal dominant condition affecting 1 in 2000 people. The deficiency is either:

- Type I (decreased quantity), or
- Type II (reduced biological activity).

Heterozygotes have 40–50% of normal plasma AT levels; homozygosity is lethal. Most patients with AT deficiency experience a thrombotic episode before the age of 50 years. Thrombosis might be severe and recurrent and these patients might have to have their blood anticoagulated with warfarin long term (see also p. 71).

Deficiencies of proteins C and S

Inheritance for both protein C and protein S deficiencies is autosomal dominant. Protein S deficiency is clinically indistinguishable from protein C deficiency. As with AT deficiency, they can be type I (decreased quantity) or type II (reduced biological activity). Heterozygotes have 50% of normal levels of protein C or S. Clinical features are similar to AT deficiency, but the thrombotic risk is four times lower. Homozygous protein C deficiency has been described where individuals have less than 1% of normal levels of protein C and have very severe disease, often presenting with problems at birth.

Defective fibrinolysis

Abnormal plasminogen and fibrinogen have been associated with reduced fibrinolytic activity and a tendency of blood to clot.

Prothrombin allele G20210A

Between 2% and 3% of the population have this prothrombin variant, which increases prothrombin levels and the thrombotic risk.

Hyperhomocysteinaemia

High levels of plasma homocysteine increase the risk of venous and arterial thrombosis.

Secondary (acquired) thrombophilia

The following conditions are associated with an increased incidence of thrombosis:

- Prolonged immobilization of the patient (venous stasis)
- Disseminated cancer (secretion of tumour substances that activate FX)
- Oestrogen therapy (increased plasma levels of factors II, VII, IX and X, and reduced levels of AT and tPA)
- Myeloproliferative disorders
- Sickle-cell anaemia
- The antiphospholipid antibody syndrome (lupus anticoagulant syndrome). This disorder is characterized by the presence of antiphospholipid antibodies in association with a clinical event. The main features of this syndrome are arterial or venous thrombosis or complications in pregnancy such as recurrent miscarriage. The disease can be idiopathic or secondary to other autoimmune disorders such as SLE.

Venous thromboembolism (VTE)

Deep vein thrombosis (DVT) occurs most commonly in the lower limbs. Symptoms and signs include:

- Swelling (usually asymmetrical)
- Pain (especially on dorsiflexion)
- Erythema.

If part of a DVT dislodges to form an embolus, this can lodge in the vasculature of the lung, a so-called pulmonary embolism (PE). PE can present most severely as collapse but symptoms often include:

- Dyspnoea
- Tachypnoea
- Pleuritic chest pain.

Well's criteria are used to evaluate the probability of VTE. A normal D-dimer level is useful to exclude VTE but may be raised in many conditions. Doppler ultrasound is used to diagnose thrombosis and a V/Q scan or spiral CT for PE.

Anticoagulation

The main use of anticoagulants is to prevent unwanted thrombus formation or extension. They act on the clotting cascade to prevent fibrin formation. Anticoagulants do not prevent platelet plug formation, nor do they break down those which are already formed.

There are two commonly used anticoagulants: heparin and warfarin. A summary of the attributes of heparin and warfarin is given in Figure 6.16.

The type of anticoagulant and the duration of its use will depend on the indication for treatment. Indications for anticoagulation therapy include:

- Prophylaxis: mechanical prosthetic heart valves, atrial fibrillation, following surgery, unstable angina
- Post-thromboembolic event: DVT, PE, acute peripheral arterial occlusion, management of MI
- During therapeutic procedures: cardiopulmonary bypass, haemodialysis.

The danger of using anticoagulants is the risk of haemorrhage. Patients already at risk of bleeding, e.g. those with peptic ulcers, oesophageal varices or severe hypertension, are contraindicated for anticoagulation. People given anticoagulants should be monitored closely to ensure the correct dose is being administered.

Fig. 6.16 Features of heparin and warfarin

	Heparin (unfractionated)	Low-molecular-weight heparin (LMWH)	Warfarin
Site of action	Potentiates antithrombin leading to inhibition of thrombin and Factor Xa	Potentiates antithrombin leading to inhibition of thrombin and Factor Xa	Inhibits vitamin K reductase
Route of administration	Subcutaneous/intravenous	Subcutaneous	Oral
Prothrombin time	Mildly prolonged	Normal	Prolonged
Activated partial thromboplastin time	Prolonged. Used for monitoring	Mildly prolonged. No use for monitoring	Prolonged
Thrombin time	Prolonged	Very mildly prolonged at therapeutic levels	Normal

Warfarin

Warfarin is a vitamin K antagonist and will, therefore, reduce the activity of vitamin-K-dependent factors. It affects the factors in the order VII, IX, X and II due to their half-lives. Proteins C and S are also inactivated by warfarin. This occurs before thrombin inactivation causing a relative deficiency in proteins C and S, which can lead to skin necrosis due to extensive thrombosis of the microvasculature within the subcutaneous fat. Because warfarin acts primarily on the extrinsic pathway, the prothrombin time is used to monitor the effect on clotting (given as INR). The target INR for different indications is given in Figure 6.17.

Fig. 6.17 Target international normalized ratio (INR) for different indications of warfarin therapy

Indication	Target INR
DVT prophylaxis	2.5
Treatment of DVT/PE	2.5
Recurrent DVT/PE (on warfarin)	3.5
Atrial fibrillation	2.5
Dilated cardiomyopathy	2.5
Mural thrombus post MI	2.5
Rheumatic mitral valve disease	2.5
Mechanical heart valve	3.0 (aortic valve) 3.5 (mitral valve)

All targets are ±0.5 i.e. a target of 2.5 means a range of 2–3. *DVT, deep vein thrombosis; MI, myocardial infarction; PE, pulmonary embolus.*

HINTS AND TIPS

The international normalized ratio (INR) is the patient's prothrombin time (PT) divided by the normal PT, with a correction factor for reagent and instrument variability. The normal range for the INR is between 0.8 and 1.2. A high INR signifies a longer PT, and therefore greater bleeding risk.

Care must be taken when using warfarin. It is teratogenic and, therefore, should not be used in early pregnancy (heparin does not cross the placenta and so can be used in pregnancy). Warfarin interacts with many drugs. Common interactions are shown in Figure 6.18.

Warfarin is potentiated in liver disease. Because warfarin has a half-life of 40 hours, the effects of changes in dose can take 4–5 days to become evident. If there is a warfarin overdose, i.e. the INR exceeds 4.5, warfarin should be stopped for 1 or 2 days and recommenced

Fig. 6.18 Common drug interactions with warfarin

Increase anticoagulant effect	Decrease anticoagulant effect
Sulphonamides Metronidazole Cephalosporins Tricyclic antidepressants Thyroxine Amiodarone High-dose salicylates (aspirin) Excess paracetamol Alcohol	Barbiturates Rifampicin Oral contraceptives Antifungals Antiepileptics (e.g. carbamazepine)

at a lower dose. The specific antidote to warfarin is vitamin K, which can be administered orally or intravenously. If the overdose has resulted in severe bleeding, prothrombin complex concentrate (PCC) should be used.

Heparin

Heparin is a glycosaminoglycan that potentiates the actions of AT. Standard (unfractionated) heparin contains molecules ranging in weight from 5000 to 30,000 kDa. The different chain lengths affect both activity and clearance, with the larger molecules being cleared more quickly. The activated partial thromboplastin time (APTT) is used to monitor unfractionated heparin therapy. Low-molecular-weight heparin (LMWH) has a mean molecular weight of 5000 kDa. LMWH is monitored only in renal failure and pregnancy. Monitoring is with an anti-Xa assay. LMWH differs from standard heparin because:

- It has greater activity against FXa than thrombin
- It has reduced protein binding and clearance
- Interactions with platelets are reduced.

LMWHs are commonly used, as subcutaneous injection, in the acute management of DVT and PE. Warfarin therapy is often started within 2 days and heparin stopped when the INR is > 2.0. LMWH is the anticoagulant of choice for prophylaxis against venous thrombosis following surgery and is increasingly used as a prophylactic against DVT in non-surgical patients.

Long-term unfractionated heparin therapy can result in osteoporosis. Other complications include bleeding and heparin-induced thrombocytopenia (HIT), which is a rare but serious problem. The risk of complications is less for LMWH than for unfractionated heparin.

Thromboprophylaxis

Hospital inpatients and patients undergoing surgery (especially obstetric and orthopaedic) are at a higher risk of VTE. Hospitals now require a VTE assessment of all inpatients, taking into account mobility and comorbidities. Strategies to prevent VTEs include good hydration, early mobilization, compression stockings and LMWH.

Therapeutic fibrinolysis

If a clot does occur fibrinolytic agents can be used. Fibrinolytics are used in a life-threatening VTE, PE, MI and CVA. They attempt to restore blood supply to an area of the circulation that has been occluded by a fibrin clot. There are different fibrinolytic agents available:

- Streptokinase: derived from group A β-haemolytic streptococci. It binds to plasminogen to form a complex that can activate other plasminogen molecules. It is highly antigenic
- Urokinase: derived from human kidney cells. It is a tPA originally isolated in urine
- Recombinant tPA: synthesized from human cells. It is highly specific for plasminogen and has a short half-life of 2–6 minutes.

Blood transfusion

Objectives

You should be able to:
- Describe what a blood transfusion is, and how and when different blood products are used
- Discuss the principles of ABO and rhesus antigens
- Explain the process of cross-matching and its importance
- Understand the dangers involved in blood transfusion.

INTRODUCTION IN BLOOD PRODUCTS

In the UK, donated blood comes from healthy volunteers between the ages of 17 and 65 (for the first donation). All donors must fill out a health questionnaire to reduce the transmission of infections. The health questionnaire includes questions about their medical history, previous blood transfusions, travel history and past behaviour associated with serious sexually transmitted infections. If a patient is deemed fit to donate, they normally have 470 mL of whole blood taken from a large vein in the antecubital fossa of the arm. The whole process normally takes less than 30 minutes. Donors have to wait 16 weeks before donating blood again.

Whole blood is very rarely given to patients. It is reserved for complex cases, and is only available if it is prearranged with the local transfusion centre. Instead, blood products are used. These include:

- Packed red cells
- Platelets
- Fresh frozen plasma
- Individual clotting factors
- Cryoprecipitate
- Albumin.

The term blood transfusion almost always indicates a transfusion of red cells.

HINTS AND TIPS

Red cells are separated from plasma and platelets and 'packed' with saline-adenine-glucose-mannitol (SAGM) solution. These packed red cells have a shelf-life of around 35 days.

INDICATIONS FOR RED CELL TRANSFUSION

Indications for blood transfusion include:

- Trauma
- Surgery
- Shock
- Severe anaemia, e.g. that associated with haemoglobinopathies
- Chemotherapy.

Some individuals do not wish to receive another person's blood, either as a result of religious beliefs or because they wish to avoid the risks associated with blood transfusion. The alternatives to blood transfusion include:

- Volume expanders: used in the acute setting to avoid the onset of shock
- Growth factors (EPO): are not used in the acute situation; they work by stimulating the bone marrow to produce more red blood cells (RBCs)
- Intraoperative blood salvage: blood lost during surgery is collected and reinfused into the patient
- Autologous blood donation: an individual donates their own blood that can be saved and infused back into the individual should they need it. This has been used for fit patients having planned surgery. Cheating athletes sometimes use this to aid their performance, a process called blood doping, as it is hard to test for
- Synthetic blood substitutes: have not yet been fully achieved; haemoglobin-based oxygen carriers and perfluorochemical compounds can perform some red cell function, but nothing has been developed yet to fully replace blood.

The main concern when administering a blood transfusion is the avoidance of an adverse immunological reaction as a result of an incompatibility between donor and recipient blood. Adverse immunological reactions occur because there are a variety of antigens on the surface of red cells. Thus, when an individual is exposed to red blood cells with different antigens (to which they are therefore not self-tolerant), they are attacked by the immune system. The resultant reactions can be severe and life-threatening.

RED-CELL ANTIGENS

The surfaces of red cells are covered with antigenic molecules. Over 400 different groups of antigens have been identified, although only some of these are clinically important in blood transfusion.

ABO antigens

The ABO system consists of three allelic genes, A, B and O, which code for sugar-residue transferase enzymes. The ABO antigen, known as the H antigen, is a glycoprotein or glycolipid with a terminal L-fructose:

- The O gene is amorphous, i.e. it has no effect on antigenic structure and leaves antigen H unchanged
- The group A gene product adds *N*-acetyl galactosamine to the H antigen
- The group B gene product adds the sugar D-galactose.

The ABO gene has three alleles, corresponding to the three antigens. Genes coding for A and B antigens are both co-dominant. Inheritance of the three ABO alleles can lead to six different genotypes and four possible phenotypes (Fig. 7.1).

By 6 months of age, the immune system will have been exposed to A- and B-like antigens in intestinal bacteria and food substances. IgM antibodies develop against A and/or B antigens, unless these antigens are present on red cells (self-tolerance). Therefore, individuals with neither A or B red-cell antigens (group O) will have both anti-A and anti-B antibodies. Those with both A and B red-cell antigens (group AB) will have neither antibody.

Fig. 7.1 ABO blood groups

Phenotype/red-cell antigens	Genotype	Antibodies
O (44%)	OO	Anti-A and anti-B
A (42%)	AO or AA	Anti-B
B (10%)	BO or BB	Anti-A
AB (4%)	AB	None

Percentages indicate the prevalence in the UK population.

Transfused blood must be ABO-compatible with the recipient's blood, otherwise recipient antibody will cause agglutination and haemolysis of the transfused cells. For example, if group A red cells are given to a group O recipient, anti-A antibodies in the recipient's serum will destroy the donor cells.

Ideally, ABO-identical blood is used; however, if this is not possible, compatible blood can be used. Blood cells of group O are not affected by anti-A or anti-B antibodies and can, therefore, be given to patients of any blood group. Consequently, blood group O is referred to as the universal donor, although it should be borne in mind that the serum of individuals with group O blood will contain anti-A and anti-B antibodies. It is always more desirable to use group-specific red cells for transfusion. Conversely, AB individuals are universal recipients because they do not possess anti-ABO antibodies and can receive blood of any ABO type.

Rhesus antigens

Rhesus (Rh) antigens are stronger immunogens and the antibodies generated are clinically important.

They are known as C, D and E, but the D antigen is the most important clinically; it is the D antigen that is referred to when describing someone as 'rhesus positive' or 'rhesus negative'. D antigen is the strongest immunogen.

The D antigen is coded for by the RhD gene. The presence of just one RhD allele (written as 'D') results in the D antigen being present. The lack of a RhD gene is written as 'd'. Thus, Rh positive individuals are DD or Dd, Rh negative individuals are dd. Approximately 85% of Caucasians are Rh positive and 15% are Rh negative. Interestingly, only 1% of individuals from Asia, and even fewer people of African origin, are Rh negative.

Anti-D antibodies are only generated when a Rh negative individual is exposed to Rh positive red cells following transfusion or pregnancy. All anti-D antibodies are IgG. Approximately 70% of Rh negative individuals produce anti-D antibodies after receiving Rh positive blood and they will develop transfusion reactions when re-transfused with Rh positive blood. As well as D positive individuals, those with C, c and E antigens may have a haemolytic reaction after transfusion, which is usually delayed rather than immediate.

RhD haemolytic disease of the newborn

If blood from a Rh positive fetus enters the circulation of an Rh negative mother, alloimmunization can occur. Small amounts of fetal blood are transferred during the third trimester and at birth. Mothers develop anti-D IgG antibodies, which cross the placenta into the fetal circulation during the course of the second pregnancy. If the second fetus is Rh positive, the IgG antibodies induce immune haemolysis of fetal red cells, which can result in hydrops fetalis.

Prevention of RhD haemolytic disease of the newborn

Passive immunization is used to prevent maternal anti-D antibody production. Therefore, all Rh negative pregnant women are given an intramuscular injection of anti-D IgG at 28 weeks' gestation (and sometimes 34 weeks depending on the preparation). If a Rh negative mother gives birth to a Rh positive child she should recieve another dose within 72 hours of the birth. The injected antibody coats Rh positive fetal red blood cells, which are removed by the reticuloendothelial system (RES) before the mother produces her own anti-D antibodies. Anti-D antibody should also be given to Rh negative mothers after all 'sensitising events', including abortions, ectopic pregnancies and amniocentesis.

HINTS AND TIPS

Red-cell antigens other than rhesus D, such as C, Kell and ABO incompatibility, can also cause haemolytic disease of the newborn. ABO incompatibility may lead to anaemia and jaundice in the newborn. It is usually short-lived and rarely requires therapy.

Other red-cell antigens

Other red-cell antigens include:

- P
- Lewis
- I
- MN
- Kell
- Duffy
- Kidd.

CROSS-MATCHING AND BLOOD TRANSFUSION

Cross-matching blood

It is important to correctly identify the patient and to label samples accurately before blood transfusions to prevent potentially fatal transfusion reactions. Cross-matching has three stages:

1. Blood grouping (ABO and Rh) of the recipient
2. Screening for abnormal recipient antibodies
   - Indirect antiglobulin test: the recipient's serum is tested against a standard pool of red cells to detect antibodies to blood group antigens other than those of the ABO and Rh systems
   - Screening cells and cell panels (to identify the antigen against which the antibody is reacting)
3. Each unit of donor blood to be transfused is then tested against the patient's serum to identify atypical antibodies in the patient. This then makes that unit of donor blood unusable by other patients.

Cross-matching normally takes under an hour but can take longer if antibodies are present. Most hospitals will only hold cross-matched blood for 24 hours.

Another pre-transfusion test is called 'group and save'. This is used when blood is not needed immediately but may be needed in the near future. It involves testing the patient's sample and storing it for 7 days. If, in that period, the patient needs a transfusion compatible blood can be provided within 15 minutes.

Emergency transfusions

During emergency situations patients often have not had a cross-match sample taken. If a patient needs blood immediately a cross-match sample should be taken and O negative blood given. There are exceptionally rare circumstances, including the management of neonatal emergencies, where whole blood is preferable.

Filtering and warming at transfusion

Blood giving sets with filters are no longer an absolute requirement for leucodepletion as donor blood is leucodepleted at the transfusion centre; however, filters are still used to help avoid contamination. Blood is warmed when it is rapidly transfused to prevent vasoconstriction, which would reduce the rate of transfusion.

Dangers in the use of blood products

Transfusion reaction

Transfusion reactions occur when incompatible blood is transfused. A summary of the complications of blood transfusions is given in Figure 7.2.

HINTS AND TIPS

The most common reason for severe complications is clerical error. Therefore, the utmost care must be taken when checking the details of the patient and the blood product. At least two healthcare professionals should check the details at the bedside.

Fig. 7.2 Complications of blood transfusions

Early	Late
Haemolytic reactions (immediate/delayed) Allergic reactions to white cells, platelets or proteins (e.g. urticaria, anaphylaxis) Febrile reactions Transfusion-related acute lung injury Circulatory overload Air embolism Thrombophlebitis Hyperkalaemia Clotting abnormalities	Transfusion transmitted infection: • Viral (e.g. CMV, HIV, hepatitis) • Bacterial (e.g. *Salmonella)* • Parasites (e.g. malaria, *Toxoplasma)* Iron overload Alloimmunization (might cause rhesus haemolytic disease in the future) Graft-versus-host disease

CMV, cytomegalovirus; HIV, human immunodeficiency virus.

Haemolytic transfusion reactions

The most severe transfusion reaction, acute haemolysis, is caused by the destruction of donor red blood cells by antibodies (IgG or IgM) present in the recipient's serum. Haemolysis caused by IgM occurs immediately, reactions caused by IgG are delayed:

- Extravascular haemolysis results from incompatibilities of blood groups that produce IgG antibodies, e.g. Rh, Kell, Duffy and Kidd. Antibody-coated red blood cells are then removed by the RES
- ABO incompatibility (usually due to a clerical error) causes intravascular haemolysis when IgM antibodies fix complement. Activation of complement generates C3a and C5a, which cause vasodilatation, increased vascular permeability and neutrophil chemotaxis.

Haemolytic transfusion reaction

Haemolytic transfusion reactions are the most serious complication of blood transfusion and usually occur as a result of ABO incompatibility. Intravascular haemolysis occurs through the activation of complement with IgM, causing symptoms of:

- Dyspnoea
- Rigors
- Lumbar pain
- Flushing
- Urticaria
- Headache.

If blood is noticed in the urine, kidney failure is of immediate concern.

Release of vasoactive substances causes profound hypotension and shock, and renal tubular necrosis can cause acute renal failure. Release of tissue thromboplastin from lysed red cells can lead to disseminated intravascular coagulation (DIC). Death occurs in 15% of cases of ABO incompatibility and usually results from severe DIC or renal failure.

Extravascular haemolysis, mediated by IgG, occurs more slowly and is less severe.

Blood products and infection risk

Infections have been transmitted in blood products. To minimize infection risk, donor blood is screened for several infective agents including syphilis, hepatitis B and C, and HIV.

Detection techniques are not foolproof. For example, HIV is detected by the presence of antibodies in donor blood. HIV has been transmitted in blood products from donors who had not seroconverted at the time of donation. Blood is taken aseptically and is then leucodepleted to reduce the risk of transmission.

There is concern about the transmission of variant Creutzfeldt–Jakob disease (vCJD), with reported cases of presumed transmission of vCJD in blood products. For this reason British plasma is no longer used in the treatment of congenital bleeding disorders.

Iron overload

The levels of iron in the body are usually controlled by the regulation of absorption. There are no physiological mechanisms to eliminate iron from the body. When people receive multiple blood transfusions, the excess iron is deposited in, and causes damage to, the heart, liver and endocrine organs. Iron-chelating agents, such as desferrioxamine and deferiprone, facilitate iron excretion.

HINTS AND TIPS

Massive transfusions are not firmly defined but one common definition is:

- Transfusing more than a patient's entire blood volume (or more than 10 units of red cells) in 24 hours.

As packed red cells are deficient in platelets and clotting factors V and VIII, massive transfusions can result in coagulopathies. These patients need platelets and fresh frozen plasma. Massive transfusions can also result in acidosis and hypothermia.

Other blood products

Platelets

Platelets are stored at room temperature (on an oscillating tray to prevent clumping) and have a half-life of 4–5 days. They can be obtained from a pool of 6–10 blood donors or from a single donor via apheresis. Indications for platelet transfusion include:

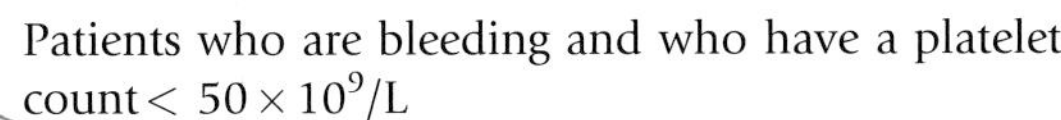

- Patients who are bleeding and who have a platelet count $< 50 \times 10^9$/L
- Following massive transfusion resulting in dilutional thrombocytopenia
- Patients with platelet dysfunction who are bleeding
- Prophylactically in patients with thrombocytopenia who are undergoing surgery or who have bone marrow failure.

Apheresis

Apheresis allows the removal of one specific component of blood such as platelets. Blood withdrawn is separated and the selected component taken out. The rest of the blood is then returned to the donor. The time this takes depends on the blood component required and is usually in the region of 1–2 hours.

Importantly, since most of the blood taken is returned, a large amount of the select component can be taken. This means that the recipient is exposed to products from fewer donors, and thus the chance of adverse reactions and infections is reduced.

Fresh-frozen plasma

Fresh-frozen plasma (FFP) contains albumin, immunoglobulins and all the clotting factors. Indications for FFP transfusion include:

- Multiple clotting factor deficiencies, e.g. severe liver disease, warfarin overdose, massive transfusion and thrombotic thrombocytopenic purpura where it is used in plasma exchange
- Specific coagulation factor replacement where no concentrate is available
- Plasma loss (albumin solution is used in many cases, e.g. burns).

HINTS AND TIPS

Compatibility of plasma is the opposite of red cells, e.g. O plasma contains anti-A and anti-B antibodies so it should only be given to O recipients.

Cryoprecipitate

Cryoprecipitate is the insoluble precipitate formed when FFP is thawed at 4°C. It contains factors VIII, vWF, factor XIII and fibrinogen, and is given to control bleeding associated with defects thereof. Cryoprecipitate can also be of use in chronic renal failure, advanced liver failure, disseminated intravascular coagulation and following massive blood transfusion.

Clotting factor concentrates

Specific clotting factor concentrates can be given to patients with clotting factor deficiencies (see Chapter 6).

White cells

Granulocyte concentrates can be given to infected neutropenic patients not responding to antibiotic therapy, but this is rare because of the risk of cytomegalovirus (CMV) transmission.

Principles of immunology

Objectives

You should be able to:

- Demonstrate a general understanding of the immune system and its interactions
- Understand the components of the innate and adaptive immune systems.

AN OVERVIEW OF IMMUNOLOGY

Learning immunology is challenging, and one of those subjects that begins to make sense after the very last lecture in the module. This is because the information received in the last lecture helps you understand the first and subsequent lectures. To help with this phenomenon we start with an overview, with the purpose of providing an understanding of immunology as a whole and building a framework in which information learned later can be stored.

The function of the immune system is to protect the body from infection and promote tissue repair following a lesion. The invaders (pathogens) range from large parasitic worms living in body cavities to small viruses that can only survive inside their host cells, with bacteria, fungi and protozoans lying somewhere in between these two extremes of size.

These pathogens and their hosts have evolved side by side, with pathogens' increasing sophistication resulting in greater evolutionary pressure for more complex immune responses.

Overview of the innate immune system

The first way the immune system protects against pathogens is to deny them entry through various physical barriers. These are the skin and mucous membranes that line the respiratory, gastrointestinal and reproductive tracts.

Once a pathogen has penetrated the body's physical defences, it is confronted by the human immune system. This system is divided into two forces, both of which get to work straight away: one responds quickly in a non-specific manner and the other occurs slowly and is specific to infecting organisms. These are the innate and adaptive immune systems, respectively. These two systems are heavily dependent on each other.

The innate immune system is composed of both cellular and soluble protein components, the most important cellular component being the phagocyte. Phagocytes are cells that engulf foreign cells and debris (phage coming from the Greek 'to eat').

Phagocytes have receptors, known as pattern recognition molecules (PRM), on their surface which sense and bind to specific molecules found on foreign cells. One important family of PRM is the toll-like receptor (TLR) family. PRMs bind to families of molecules, or ligands, which can range from carbohydrates to flagellae. For example TLR4 binds lipo-polysaccharide (endotoxin) which is a molecule found in the cell membrane of many different bacteria. Phagocytes also recognise pathogens that have been flagged by other parts of the immune system, such as complement and antibody.

There are two types of phagocyte: the macrophage and the neutrophil. The macrophage is long lived and stationed within tissues, patrolling for the presence of trespassers. Upon contact with a pathogen (e.g. a bacterium), the macrophage engulfs it, a process known as phagocytosis. The bacterium is contained inside the macrophage, within a 'phagosome' which then fuses with a lysosome that contains enzymes and chemicals that destroy the bacterium.

Macrophages secrete proteins called cytokines, the functions of which include attracting other cells (including short-lived neutrophils), increasing the permeability of the vascular endothelium and even increasing the production of neutrophils in the bone marrow.

Neutrophils act as reinforcements for the sentinel macrophages, following the trail of cytokines to the site of infection, a process called chemotaxis. Neutrophils are professional phagocytes extremely effective at killing pathogens; however, they are short lived (a failsafe to avoid excessive destruction of normal tissue) and, if the infection persists, continued secretion of cytokines will result in further mobilization of neutrophils.

> **HINTS AND TIPS**
>
> Neutrophils can be recognized histologically as they have multilobed nuclei and cytoplasmic granules.

Other important cells in the innate immune response include natural killer (NK) cells (a form of lymphocyte) and degranulating cells, such as eosinophils and mast cells.

The humoral (soluble) section of the innate immune system is complement. Complement comprises approximately 20 proteins that are activated through various pathways and can destroy pathogens directly through the formation of the membrane attack complex (MAC) or prepare (opsonize) them for destruction by other parts of the immune system.

The combination of phagocytes and complement systems is sufficient for dealing with most bacteria and fungi. However, certain pathogens have evolved to hide inside a host's cells where phagocytes and complement cannot reach them. Another problem with this early immune system is that a host can be infected with the same pathogen over and over again and the response has to start afresh each time.

> **HINTS AND TIPS**
>
> Pathogens are detected by the innate immune system in many ways, including through pattern recognition molecules (PRMs), complement opsonization and antibody binding.

Overview of the adaptive immune system

The adaptive immune system, which evolved at about the same time as the vertebrates, has developed to combat both these flaws of the innate system. This development has led to the adaptive immune system having many more receptors for pathogenic molecules, since such receptors are not fixed, but are formed through genetic recombination. This genetic recombination is the basis of the specificity of the adaptive immune system. These receptors are expressed on specialized lymphocytes called T and B cells.

T cells are able to recognize intracellular infections. This is possible as our cells evolved a method whereby the complete range of proteins within the cell is expressed as short peptides on its surface. The molecules that bind the small peptides to be expressed on the cell surface are called the major histocompatibility complex (MHC), also known as human leucocyte antigen (HLA).

Some cells are particularly good at presenting antigen to T cells. These cells are known as antigen-presenting cells (APCs), and examples are macrophages and dendritic cells. These cells are seen as the link between the innate and adaptive immune systems, in that by presenting antigen to T cells they activate an adaptive response.

One subset of T lymphocytes are called T helper (Th) cells. These cells usually express a glycoprotein called CD4, and are therefore known as $CD4^+$ T cells. These cells are crucial in determining the type of immune response deployed. Another subset of T lymphocytes are called cytotoxic T cells. They are effector cells and can destroy infected host cells. These cells usually express CD8 and are thus referred to as $CD8^+$ T cells. Activated B cells, known as plasma cells, can release their receptors into blood and bodily secretions. These free receptors are called antibodies or immunoglobulin (Ig). The function of antibody is to flag up foreign antigens for destruction by other parts of the immune system. There are five different classes of antibodies known as IgA, IgD, IgE, IgG and IgM. They all have different properties and roles.

The adaptive immune system has the capacity to 'remember' previously encountered pathogens. This memory is dependent on long-lived memory B and T cells. They enable the innate immune system to recognize and confront the pathogen if exposure is repeated. It mounts a rapid and specific response, preventing infection.

> **HINTS AND TIPS**
>
> The adaptive immune system is triggered through antigen-presenting cells (APCs). T cells coordinate the adaptive immune response, as well as eradicating some pathogens. B cells create antibody, enabling the innate immune system to recognize the pathogen, as well as be responsible for immunological memory.

Essential differences between the innate and adaptive immune systems are outlined in Figure 8.1.

Both the innate and adaptive immune systems comprise cellular and humoral components (Figure 8.2).

An overview of the body's defences against infection is shown in Figure 8.3.

Cytokines

Cytokines are small, secreted proteins and are the messengers of the immune system, allowing cells to communicate. They act locally, via specific cell-surface receptors, as part of both the innate and adaptive

Fig. 8.1 Essential differences between the innate and adaptive immune systems

Innate immune system	Adaptive immune system
Provides a rapid response It is not antigen specific The response does not improve with repeated exposure Uses germ line genes to produce pattern recognition molecules	The response takes time to develop, because: • It is specific for each different antigen • Initial exposure to an antigen leaves memory cells; subsequent infections with the same antigen are therefore dealt with more quickly Uses genetic recombination to produce receptors.

Fig. 8.2 Components of the innate and adaptive immune systems

	Innate system	Adaptive system
Cellular components	Monocytes/ macrophages Neutrophils Eosinophils Basophils Mast cells Natural killer cells	B cells/ plasma cells T cells
Secreted components	Complement Cytokines Lysozyme Acute phase proteins Interferons	Antibody Cytokines

immune response. Cytokines have many effects, but in general they stimulate the immune response through:

- Growth, activation and survival of various cells
- Increased production of surface molecules such as MHC.

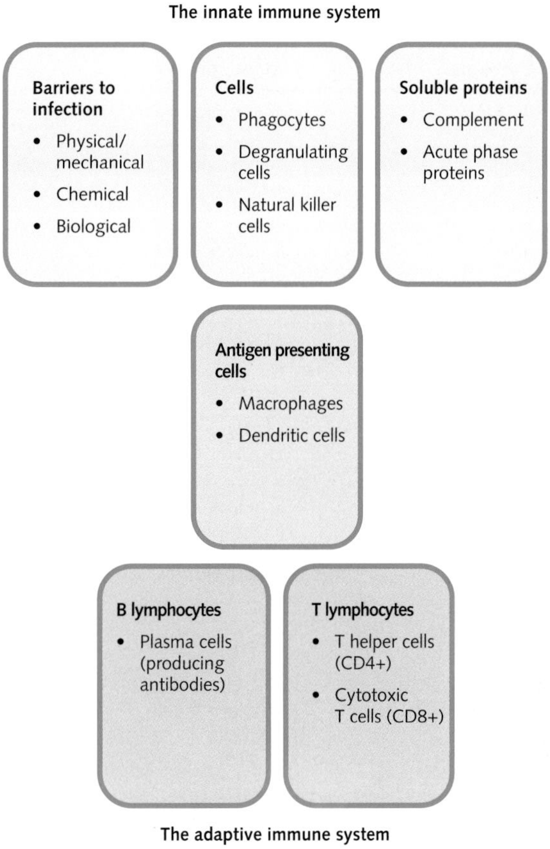

The innate immune system

Barriers to infection
- Physical/ mechanical
- Chemical
- Biological

Cells
- Phagocytes
- Degranulating cells
- Natural killer cells

Soluble proteins
- Complement
- Acute phase proteins

Antigen presenting cells
- Macrophages
- Dendritic cells

B lymphocytes
- Plasma cells (producing antibodies)

T lymphocytes
- T helper cells (CD4+)
- Cytotoxic T cells (CD8+)

The adaptive immune system

Fig. 8.3 A simple schematic of the immune system. For a pathogen to colonize human tissues, it must invade the body's barriers to infection and then evade the innate and adaptive immune systems. Antigen-presenting cells (APCs) act as the bridge between the two systems.

Important cytokines include members of the interleukin (IL) family, interferon (IFN) family and tumour necrosis factor (TNF) family. A group of cytokines are responsible for chemotaxis, a process in which leukocytes are guided to sites of infection. These cytokines are called chemokines. IL-8 is an important member of this family. These proteins are important because drugs have been designed to block their effects.

Some important cytokines and their main actions are shown in Figure 8.4.

Fig. 8.4 Important cytokines and their actions

Cytokine	Main sources	Main actions
IL-1	Macrophages	Fever T-cell and macrophage activation
IL-2	T helper 1 cells	Growth of T cells Stimulates growth of B cells and NK cells
IL-4	T helper 2 cells	Activation and growth of B cells IgG1, IgE and MHC class II induction of B cells Induces CD4 T cells to differentiate into T helper 2 cells
IL-6	Macrophages	Lymphocyte activation Increased antibody production Fever, induces acute phase proteins
IL-8	Macrophages	Chemotactic factor for neutrophils Activates neutrophils
IL-10	T helper 2 cells Macrophages	Inhibits immune function
IL-12	Macrophages	Activates NK cells Induces CD4 T cells to differentiate into T helper 1 cells
IL-17	T helper 17 cells	Proinflammatory Recruits neutrophils
Interferon-γ	T helper 1 cells NK cells	Activation of macrophages and NK cells Produces antiviral state in neighbouring cells Increases expression of MHC class I and II molecules Inhibits T helper 2 cells
TNF	T helper cells Macrophages	Activates macrophages and induces nitric oxide production Proinflammatory Fever and shock

IL, interleukin; MHC, major histocompatibility complex; NK, natural killer; TNF, tumour necrosis factor.

The innate immune system

Objectives

You should be able to:
- Explain the barriers to infection
- Understand how phagocytes kill pathogens
- Outline the complement cascade
- Describe how measurement of different components of the innate immune system can be used to diagnose different clinical scenarios.

Innate defences can be classified into three main groups:
1. Barriers to infection
2. Cells
3. Serum proteins and the complement system.

BARRIERS TO INFECTION

Physical and mechanical

Skin and mucosal membranes act as physical barriers to the entry of pathogens. Tight junctions between cells prevent the majority of pathogens from entering the body. The flushing actions of tears, saliva and urine protect epithelial surfaces from colonization. High oxygen tension in the lungs, and body temperature, can also inhibit microbial growth.

In the respiratory tract, mucus is secreted to trap microorganisms. They are then mechanically expelled by:
- Beating cilia (mucociliary escalator)
- Coughing
- Sneezing.

Chemical

The growth of microorganisms is inhibited at acidic pH (e.g. in the stomach and vagina). Lactic acid and fatty acids in sebum (produced by sebaceous glands) maintain the skin pH between 3 and 5. Enzymes such as lysozyme (found in saliva, sweat and tears) and pepsin (present in the gut) destroy microorganisms.

Biological (normal flora)

A person's normal flora is formed when non-pathogenic bacteria colonize epithelial surfaces. Normal flora protects the host by:
- Competing with pathogenic bacteria for nutrients and attachment sites
- Production of antibacterial substances.

The use of antibiotics can disrupt the normal flora, making pathogenic organisms more likely to cause disease.

CELLS OF INNATE IMMUNITY

The cells of the innate immune system consist of:
- Phagocytes
- Degranulating cells
- Natural killer cells.

Phagocytes

Phagocytes (macrophages and neutrophils) engulf and then destroy pathogens. Macrophages are long-lived sentinel cells stationed at likely sites of infection; upon infection they release cytokines that recruit the shorter-lived but more actively phagocytic neutrophils.

Neutrophils (for structure, see p. 37; for production, see p. 2)

Neutrophils comprise 50–70% of circulating white cells. Neutrophils arrive quickly at the site of inflammation and in the act of killing pathogens they die; in fact, dead neutrophils are the major constituent of pus. In response to tissue damage, chemicals released by macrophages and complement proteins, neutrophils migrate from the bloodstream to the site of the insult (see Chapter 11). They are phagocytes and have an important role in engulfing and killing extracellular pathogens. The process of phagocytosis and the mechanisms of killing are shown on page 85. During inflammation, neutrophil production is stimulated by the cytokine

G-CSF. A high neutrophil count is part of the acute phase response (see below). Neutrophils can be activated and recruited either by IL-8 and TNF secreted by macrophages, or by IL-17 secreted by T cells of the adaptive immune system.

HINTS AND TIPS

Neutropenic individuals are at an increased risk of serious bacterial infections. These patients should be treated early and aggressively to reduce the chance of sepsis.

Mononuclear phagocyte system

Monocytes and macrophages comprise the other major group of phagocytic cells. Monocytes account for 5–10% of the white cell count and circulate in the blood for approximately 8 hours before migrating into the tissues, where they differentiate into macrophages; these macrophages can live for decades. Some macrophages become adapted for specific functions in particular tissues, e.g. Kupffer cells in the liver and glial cells in the brain. Monocytes also differentiate into osteoclasts and microglial cells.

In comparison to monocytes, macrophages:

- Are larger and longer-lived
- Have greater phagocytic ability
- Have a larger repertoire of lytic enzymes and secretory products.

Macrophages phagocytose and destroy their targets using similar mechanisms to neutrophils. The rate of phagocytosis can be greatly increased by opsonins such as IgG and the complement protein C3b (neutrophils and macrophages have receptors for these molecules, which may be bound to the antigenic surface). Intracellular pathogens, e.g. *Mycobacterium*, can prove difficult for macrophages to kill. They are either resistant to destruction inside the phagosome or can enter the macrophage cytoplasm. For the immune system to act against these pathogens, T cell help is required.

In addition to phagocytosis, macrophages can secrete a number of compounds into the extracellular space, including cytokines (TNF, IL-8 and IL-1) and hydrolytic enzymes. Macrophages are also able to process and present antigen in association with class II MHC molecules.

Macrophages express a wide array of surface molecules including:

- Fc-γRI–III (receptors for the Fc portion of IgG, types I–III) and complement receptors
- Pattern recognition molecules (PRMs)
- Cytokine receptors, e.g. TNF-α and interferon-γ (IFN-γ)
- MHC and B7 molecules (to activate the adaptive immune response).

Macrophages can be activated by:

- Cytokines such as IFN-γ
- Contact with complement or products of blood coagulation
- Direct contact with the target through PRM stimulation.

Following activation, macrophages become more efficient phagocytes and have increased secretory and microbicidal activity. They also stimulate the adaptive immune system by expressing higher levels of MHC class II molecules and secreting cytokines.

In comparison to neutrophils, macrophages:

- Are longer-lived (they do not die after dealing with pathogens)
- Are larger (diameter 25–50 μm), enabling phagocytosis of larger targets
- Move and phagocytose more slowly
- Retain Golgi apparatus and rough endoplasmic reticulum and can therefore synthesize new proteins, including lysosomal enzymes and secretory products
- Can act as antigen-presenting cells (APCs).

Killing by phagocytes

The process of phagocytosis allows cells to engulf matter that needs to be destroyed. The cell can then digest the material in a controlled fashion before releasing the contents. The process of phagocytosis is shown in Figure 9.1.

Natural killer (NK) cells

NK cells utilize cell-surface receptors to identify virally modified or cancerous cells. NK cells do not require T cell help to kill pathogens, although they are more effective when T helper cells secrete IFN-γ. One set of receptors activates NK cells, initiating killing; others inhibit the cells:

- Activating receptors include calcium-binding C-lectins, which recognize certain cell-surface carbohydrates. Because these carbohydrates are present on the surface of normal host cells, a system of inhibitory receptors acts to prevent killing
- Killer inhibitor receptors (KIRs), members of the immunoglobulin gene superfamily, are specific for class I MHC molecules. Human NK cells also express an inhibitory receptor (a heterodimer CD94:NKG2) that detects non-classical class I MHC molecules.

NK cells can also destroy antibody-coated target cells irrespective of the presence of MHC molecules, a process known as antibody-dependent cell-mediated cytotoxicity. This occurs because killing is initiated by cross-linking of receptors for the Fc portion of IgG1 and IgG3.

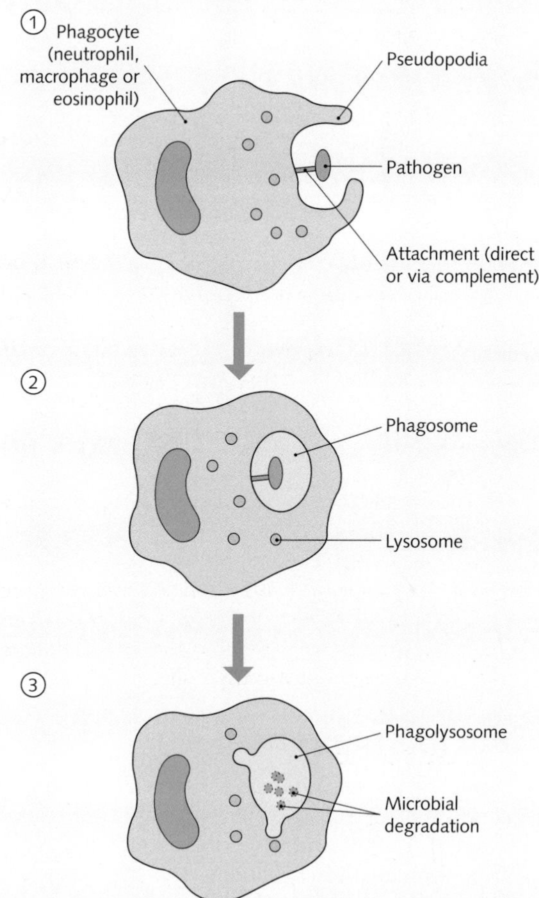

Fig. 9.1 Phagocytosis. Phagocytes sense an organism and bind it via non-specific receptors or via complement or antibody. Pseudopodia extend from the surface of the cell to surround the pathogen (1). The pseudopodia fuse around the organism, producing a vesicle known as a phagosome (2). Lysosomes fuse with the phagosome to form phagolysosomes (3). Chemicals within the lysosome, and other granules that fuse with the phagolysosome, lead to degradation of the organism. The microbial products are then released.

NK cells are not clonally restricted, have no memory and are not very specific in their action. They induce apoptosis in target cells (Fig. 9.2) by:

- Ligation of FAS or TNF receptors on the target cells (NK cells produce TNF and exhibit FASL). This initiates a sequence of caspase recruitment and activation, resulting in apoptosis
- Degranulation by NK cells, which releases perforins and granzymes. Perforin molecules insert into and polymerize within the target cell membrane. This forms a pore through which granzymes can pass. Granzyme B then initiates apoptosis from within the target cell cytoplasm.

HINTS AND TIPS

FAS receptors are found on human cells. Once they bind to the FAS ligand (FASL) they stimulate apoptosis.

Mast cells and basophils (for structure, see p. 40)

Mast cells and basophils have similar functions but are found in different locations; basophils comprise $< 1\%$ of circulating white cells, whereas mast cells are resident in the tissues.

High concentrations of mast cells are found close to blood vessels in connective tissue, skin and mucosal membranes. The two types of mast cell—mucosal and connective tissue—differ in their tissue distribution, protease content and secretory profiles.

Mast cells function by discharging their granule contents. Degranulation is triggered by cross-linking of high-affinity receptors for the Fc portion of IgE (Fig. 9.3). Cross-linkage results in an influx of calcium ions into the cell, which induces release of pharmacologically active mediators from granules (Fig. 9.4). Mast cell activation releases leukotrienes, which attract eosinophils to the site of worm infection. This plays an important role in the development of an episode of a type I hypersensitivity, with the mast cells and basophils providing the early phase response and the eosinophils mediating the late phase response. This is important in allergic responses (type I hypersensitivity reactions, see p. 117).

HINTS AND TIPS

During severe allergy (anaphylaxis, see p. 121) mast cell tryptase levels increase for a few hours. This is a useful diagnostic test for anaphylaxis.

Eosinophils (for structure, see p. 38)

Eosinophils comprise 1–3% of circulating white cells and are found principally in tissues. They are derived from the colony-forming unit for granulocytes, erythrocytes, monocytes and megakaryocytes (CFU-GEMM) haematopoietic precursor and their maturation is similar to that of the neutrophil (see p. 2). They are important in the defence against parasites and cause damage by extracellular degranulation. Their granules contain major basic protein, cationic protein, peroxidase and perforin-like molecules. The peroxidase generates hypochlorous acid, major basic protein damages the parasite's outer

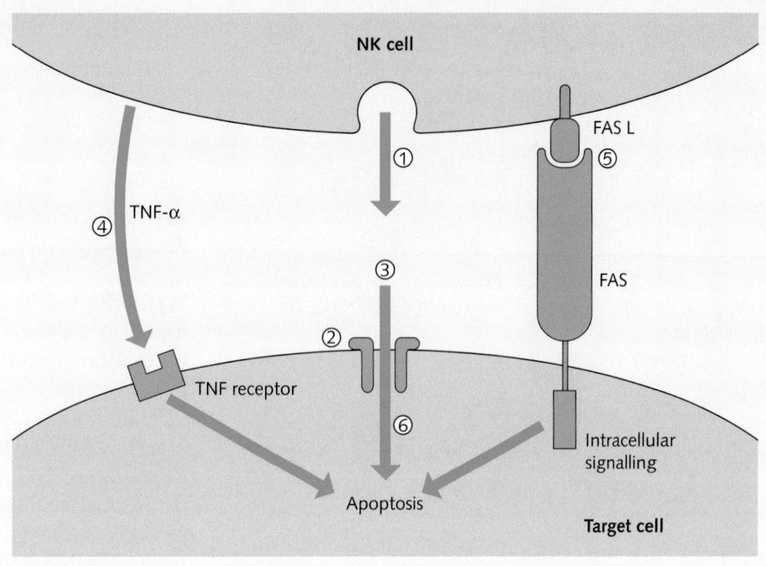

Fig. 9.2 Mechanism of killing by natural killer (NK) cells (1). Activation of NK cells in the absence of an inhibitory signal results in degranulation (2). Perforins form a pore in the target cell, allowing entry of granzymes (3). TNF produced by NK cells acts on the target's cell receptors (4). FASL interacts with target cell FAS (5). Intracellular signalling from FAS, TNF receptors and granzymes results in apoptosis (6).

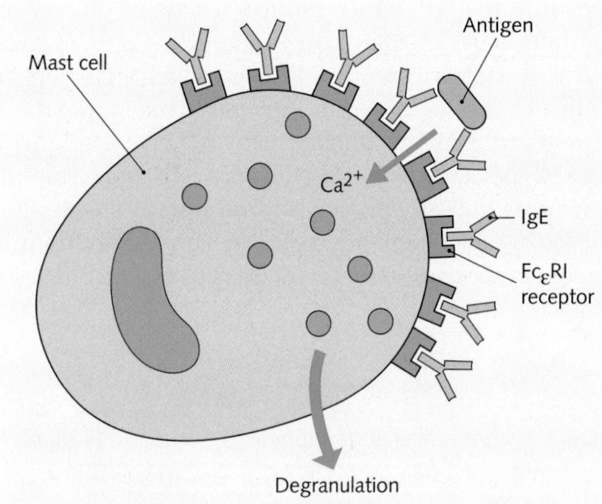

Fig. 9.3 Activation of mast cells by immunoglobulin E (IgE). IgE, produced by plasma cells, binds via its Fc domain to receptors on the mast cell surface. Cross-linking of these receptors by an antigen causes an influx of calcium ions (Ca^{2+}) into the cell. Calcium ions cause a rapid degranulation of inflammatory mediators from the mast cell.

surface (as well as host tissues) and cationic protein acts as a neurotoxin, damaging the parasite's nervous tissue.

SOLUBLE PROTEINS

The soluble proteins that contribute to innate immunity (Fig. 9.5) can be divided into antimicrobial serum agents and proteins produced by cells of the immune system.

Acute phase proteins

The acute phase response is a systemic reaction to infection or tissue injury, where macrophages release cytokines IL-1, IL-6 and TNF; these cytokines reach the liver through the circulation. The liver responds by increasing its production of certain plasma proteins. These so-named acute phase proteins (APPs) are:

- C-reactive protein
- Serum amyloid A
- Complement components
- Fibrinogen
- α_1-Antitrypsin
- Caeruloplasmin
- Haptoglobulin.

The change in plasma concentration is accompanied by fever, leucocytosis, thrombocytosis, catabolism of muscle proteins and fat deposits. Synthesis of APPs is enhanced by cytokines secreted by macrophages and endothelial cells. The two main APPs are C-reactive protein (CRP) and serum amyloid A (SAA).

The extent of the rise in the plasma concentration of different APPs varies:

- Increased 50% above normal levels: caeruloplasmin
- Increased several fold above normal levels: α_1-glycoprotein, α_1-proteinase inhibitor, haptoglobulin, fibrinogen
- 100–1000-fold increase: CRP, SAA.

The concentration of other plasma proteins, most notably albumin and transferrin, falls.

Fig. 9.4 Mast cell mediators and their actions

Mediator			Action
Primary	Histamine		Increased capillary permeability, vasodilatation, smooth muscle contraction
	Serotonin		Increased capillary permeability, vasodilatation, smooth muscle contraction, platelet aggregation
	Heparin		Anticoagulation (see p. 72), modulates tryptase
	Proteases	Tryptase	Activates complement (C3)
		Chymase	Increased mucus secretion
	Platelet-activating factor		Platelet aggregation and activation, increased capillary permeability, vasodilatation, chemotactic for leucocytes, neutrophil activation
Secondary	Leukotrienes (C_4, D_4, B_4)		Vasodilatation, smooth muscle contraction, mucus secretion, chemotactic for neutrophils
	Prostaglandins (D_2)		Vasodilatation, smooth muscle contraction, chemotactic for neutrophils, potentiation of other mediators
	Bradykinin		Increased capillary permeability, vasodilatation, smooth muscle contraction, stimulation of pain nerve endings
	Cytokines		Various

Mast cells contain many preformed (primary) mediators that are stored in granules. They can also synthesize new (secondary) mediators when they are activated.

Fig. 9.5 The soluble proteins of innate immunity

	Protein	Notes
Secreted agents	Lysozyme	Bactericidal enzyme in mucus, saliva, tears, sweat and breast milk Cleaves peptidoglycan in the cell wall
Innate antimicrobial serum agents	Lactoferrin	Iron-binding protein that competes with microorganisms for iron, an essential metabolite
	Complement	Group of ~20 proenzymes Activation leads to an enzyme cascade, the products of which enhance phagocytosis and mediate cell lysis Alternative pathway can be activated by non-specific mechanism
	Mannan-binding lectin	Activates the complement system
	C-reactive protein	Acute phase protein, produced by the liver Serum concentration rises > 100-fold in inflammation, for example infection and following infarction Binds C-polysaccharide cell wall component of bacteria and fungi Activates complement via classical pathway Opsonizes for phagocytosis
Proteins produced by cells of the innate system	Interferon-α Interferon-β	Produced by virally infected cells Induces a state of viral resistance in neighbouring cells by: • Inducing genes that will destroy viral DNA • Inducing MHC class I expression
	Interferon-γ	Mainly produced by activated NK cells Activates NK cells and macrophages

MHC, major histocompatibility complex; NK, natural killer.

C-reactive protein

Levels of CRP rise within hours of tissue injury or infection. The actions of CRP are outlined in Figure 9.5. CRP elevation can be slight (e.g. cerebrovascular accident), moderate (e.g. myocardial infarction) or marked (e.g. bacterial infections).

HINTS AND TIPS

TNF-α, IL-1 and IL-6 released by macrophages stimulate the liver to produce the acute phase proteins.

Serum amyloid A

SAA levels rise within hours of tissue injury or infection. SAA induces the migration of inflammatory cells to sites of inflammation and functions as an opsonin, particularly against Gram-negative bacteria. Persistent elevation of SAA can lead to its deposition in tissues in amyloidosis (see p. 54).

Erythrocyte sedimentation rate

The erythrocyte sedimentation rate (ESR) is an index of the acute phase response. It is especially representative of the concentration of fibrinogen and α-globulins. Elevated fibrinogen levels cause red cells to form stacks (rouleaux), which sediment more rapidly than individual blood cells.

HINTS AND TIPS

In chronic inflammation, high C-reactive protein (CRP) and erythrocyte sedimentation rate (ESR) persist. The resulting catabolism of muscle and fat may lead to severe weight loss.

The acute phase response

The acute phase response provides us with chemical markers of inflammation that can be measured. In a child presenting with abdominal pain a C-reactive protein (CRP) can aid the clinician in their diagnosis. A normal CRP can allow more conservative management whereas a raised CRP would indicate an inflammatory response and necessitate urgent treatment, such as surgery in differentiating the abdominal pain in constipation from that of appendicitis.

The neutrophil count and erythrocyte sedimentation rate (ESR) take more time than CRP to become elevated. They are a useful marker measured in chronic inflammatory diseases. Some hospitals now measure plasma viscosity instead of ESR. However, ESR levels are still crucial for the diagnosis of giant cell (temporal) arteritis.

The complement system

The complement system (so-called because its actions are *complementary* to the function of antibody) is, in fact, much older in evolutionary terms than antibody and is equally important.

Complement is a collection of over 20 serum proteins that are always at high levels in the blood of the healthy individual. The complement system may seem complex with all the alphanumerical naming and active and inactive components. Thinking about it simply, it is a system that has three methods of activating a common pathway, which in turn has three results or effectors. The reason for the large number of proteins is to allow amplification; many of the components of complement are proenzymes that, when cleaved, activate more complement.

The three pathways that activate the complement system are the classical, the alternative and the lectin. All pathways result in the activation of the complement component C3 to C3 convertase. An overview of the complement system is given in Figure 9.6.

The classical pathway

The classical pathway was discovered first and involves the activation of complement by the Fc portion of antibody. IgM is particularly good at activating complement as it is a pentamer (has five Fc portions):

- Fc activates C1
- C1 activates C2 and C4
- C2 and C4 activate C3 (C3 convertase).

The alternative pathway

C3 is an unstable molecule and without inhibition spontaneously breaks down to the very reactive C3b; C3b reacts to two common chemical functional groups, the amino and hydroxyl groups. C3b is therefore neutralized quickly by water. However, with many pathogens made up of proteins and carbohydrates that contain these functional groups, C3b attaches to the pathogen and is not broken down. C3b then reacts with more complement components to form C3bBb; this is C3 convertase.

The lectin pathway

Mannan-binding lectin (MBL), which is normally found in serum, binds to MBL-associated serine proteases (MASP). This complex bears structural homology to the C1 complex. When MBL binds to carbohydrate on the surface of bacteria, MASP is activated. MASP then acts on C4 and C2 to generate the C3 convertase of the classical pathway.

C3 convertase

With the production of C3 convertase, all three pathways converge. C3 convertase has enzymatic effects against C3 and enables the production of large quantities of C3b, thus producing a major amplification step in the complement pathway.

Effectors of complement

C5 is cleaved into C5a and C5b. C5b then triggers the activation of C6–C9. These form the membrane attack complex (MAC). The MAC attacks pathogens by inserting a hole in their cell membrane; the pathogen then

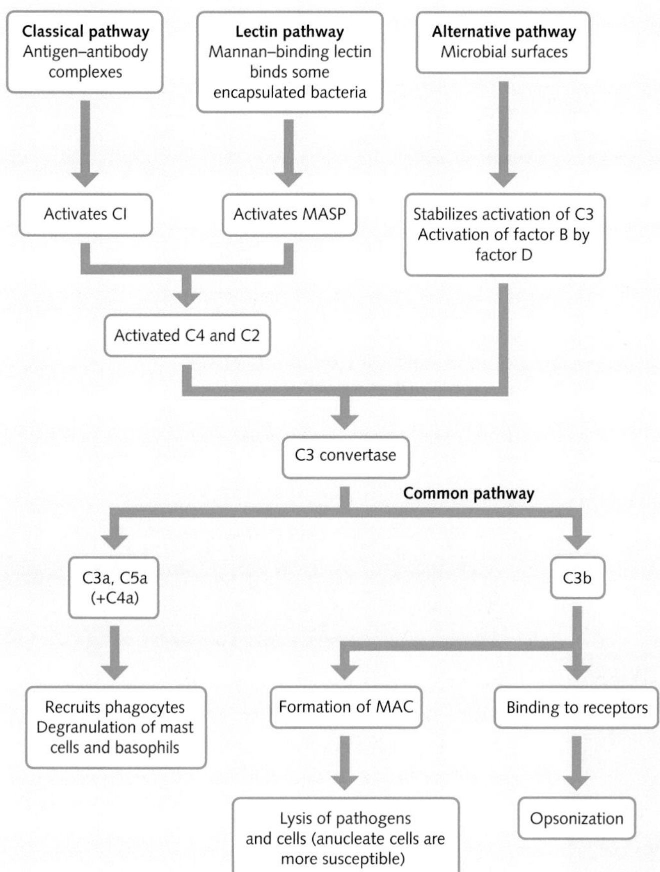

Fig. 9.6 Overview of the complement system. Cell lysis by complement is due to formation of the membrane attack complex (MAC). This is formed when C5b, C6, C7, C8 and C9 bind together to form a 10-nm pore in the cell surface. MASP, mannan-binding lectin associated serine protease.

dies via osmotic lysis. The MAC appears to be the only way the immune system has of killing one family of bacteria, the *Neisseria* (a family that includes meningococcus and gonococcus).

The cleaved fragments C3a and C5a are anaphylotoxins which are chemoattractant for other immune cells which follow the concentration gradient to the infection. Complement also opsonizes bacteria as macrophages have receptors for C3b.

These functions are summarized in Figure 9.7.

Inhibitors of complement

As we have seen, complement can activate spontaneously through the alternative pathway. Complement is regulated by inhibitory molecules which are necessary to prevent complement-mediated damage of healthy cells. There are nine complement inhibitors which act at various levels throughout the pathway:

- Membrane cofactor protein, complement receptor type 1, C4b-binding protein and factor H: these prevent assembly of C3 convertase
- Decay accelerating factor: this accelerates decay of C3 convertase
- C1 inhibitor: inhibits C1
- Factor I and membrane cofactor protein: cleave C3b and C4b
- CD59 (protectin): prevents the formation of the membrane attack complex (MAC).

Hereditary angioedema

Deficiency in even one of these inhibitory components can result in significant disease. For example, deficiency in C1 inhibitor results in hereditary angioedema (HAE; see Fig. 9.8) types I and II, conditions where there is activation of the classical pathway with minimal stimulation. This is of particular significance if the stimulation is in the larynx as it can lead to uncontrolled swelling. This laryngeal oedema can obstruct the airway and without infusion of C1 inhibitor can prove fatal. The clinical picture resembles anaphylaxis (see Chapter 12) and patients are often treated with adrenaline, which has no effect.

Fig. 9.7 Functions of complement

Function	Notes
Cell lysis	Insertion of MAC causes lysis of Gram-negative bacteria Nucleated cells are more resistant to lysis because they endocytose MAC
Inflammation	C3a, C4a, C5a cause degranulation of mast cells and basophils C3a and C5a are chemotactic for neutrophils
Opsonization	Phagocytes have C3b receptors, which means phagocytosis is enhanced when pathogens are coated in C3b
Solubilization and clearance of immune complexes	Complement prevents immune complex precipitation and solubilizes complexes that have already been precipitated Complexes coated in C3b bind to CR1 on red blood cells The complexes are then removed in the spleen

MAC, membrane attack complex.

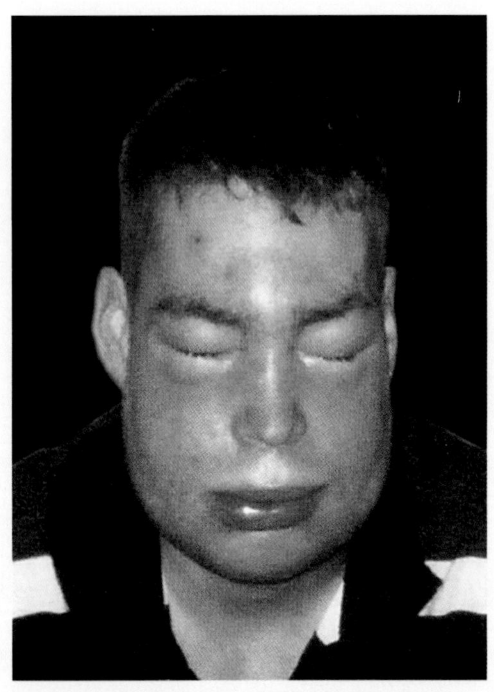

Fig. 9.8 A patient with hereditary angioedema.

INNATE IMMUNE SYSTEM PATTERN RECOGNITION MOLECULES

We have already come across the recognition molecules MBL and C1q in the complement system. These are found in solution in the serum and are classified as collectins, being composed of collagen-like and lectin portions. Lectins are any protein that binds sugar molecules, usually on the surface of bacteria, e.g. MBL binds to the sugar mannose.

NOD is a pattern recognition molecule with some special characteristics. It recognizes bacterial cell wall components and stimulates an immune response. The NOD gene is mutated in some individuals with Crohn's disease.

Toll-like receptors (TLRs) are a family of about a dozen pattern recognition molecules. When they bind their lectin, they send a signal to innate immune system cells which then secrete cytokines. They have a few important clinical roles. In endotoxic shock (septic shock) TLR-4 is stimulated by vast amounts of LPS released during septicaemia. This causes release of TNF, which in turn activates nitrous oxide synthase causing a fall in blood pressure.

Drugs designed to bind and stimulate TLRs are being used in situations where it is helpful to stimulate a more powerful immune response, for example in some vaccines and cancer treatments.

The adaptive immune system

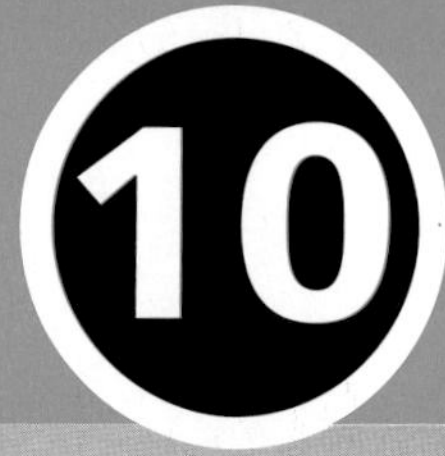

Objectives

You should be able to:

- Understand the structure and function of the major histocompatibility complex MHC
- Understand the principle of genetic recombination, and how this leads to receptor diversity
- Explain the functions of the differing classes of immunoglobulins
- Draw the structure and understand the functions of immunoglobulins and T cell receptors
- Understand the differences in the types of T helper cells and the immune responses they evoke.

THE IMMUNOGLOBULIN DOMAIN

B and T cell surface receptors are members of the immunoglobulin gene superfamily. Genes in this family code for proteins composed of motifs called immunoglobulin (Ig) domains. All molecules in the immunoglobulin superfamily extend from the surface of cells. They are flexible and include specialist domains; the antigen receptor site on B cell receptors is an example.

Members of this gene family include:

- Immunoglobulin (B cell receptor)
- T cell receptor
- MHC molecules
- T cell accessory molecules such as CD4
- Certain adhesion molecules, e.g. ICAM-1, ICAM-2 and VCAM-1.

Each domain is approximately 110 amino acids in length. The polypeptide chain in each domain is folded into seven or eight antiparallel beta strands. The strands are arranged to form two opposing sheets, linked by a disulphide bond and hydrophobic interactions. This compact structure is called the immunoglobulin fold.

Structure of B and T cell surface antigen receptors

Structure of immunoglobulin

The B cell surface receptor is a membrane-bound immunoglobulin (mIg) molecule. mIg recognizes the conformational structure (shape) of antigenic epitopes. Ig is composed of two light and two heavy chains. In the B cell receptor (Fig. 10.1), mIg associates with two Ig-α/Ig-β dimers (members of the immunoglobulin gene superfamily). Signal transduction through the mIg is thought to be mediated by the Ig-α/Ig-β heterodimers.

Ig is also secreted by plasma cells (see p. 98). The extracellular portion of mIg is identical in structure to secretory Ig. mIg differs from secreted Ig (sIg) because it has transmembrane and cytoplasmic portions that anchor it to the membrane. Different Ig classes can be expressed on the same B cell and may indicate the stage of development of the B cell, e.g. a mature, but antigenically unchallenged B cell expresses both mIgM and mIgD. The antigenic specificity of all of the mIg molecules expressed on any given B cell is the same.

Antigen recognition by T cells differs from antigen recognition by B cells:

- T cells recognize peptide fragments of an antigen in association with MHC molecules; these fragments of antigen are processed by APCs before they are presented to the T cell
- T cells recognize antigen only when it is associated with a molecule of the MHC.

The T cell surface antigen receptor consists of the T cell receptor (TCR) associated with CD3. The TCR is a heterodimer, comprising α- and β-chains, or γ-and δ-chains. Approximately 95% of T cells express αβ-receptors. The TCR is structurally similar to the immunoglobulin Fab region (see p. 97). Each chain comprises two immunoglobulin domains, one variable and one constant, linked by a disulphide bond. As in the variable domains of immunoglobulin, three variable regions on each chain combine to form the antigen-binding site.

CD3 is made up of three polypeptide dimers, consisting of four or five different peptide chains. The dimers are γε, δε and ζζ (found in 90% of CD3 molecules) or ζη. The γ-, δ- and ε-chains are members of the Ig gene superfamily. The TCR recognizes and binds antigen, and CD3, functionally analogous to the Ig-α/Ig-β heterodimer in B cells, is involved in signal transduction (Fig. 10.2).

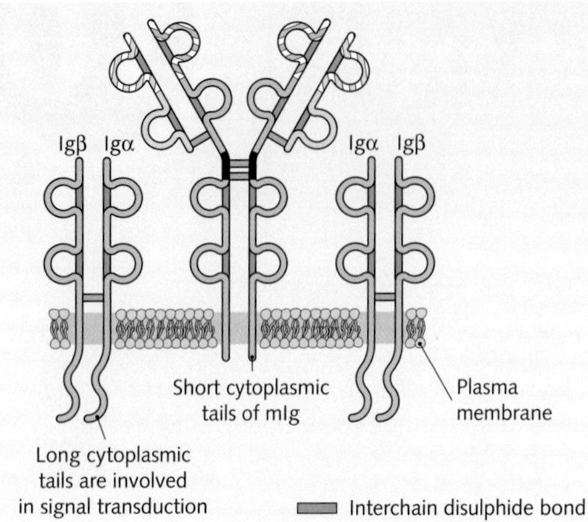

Fig. 10.1 Structure of the B cell surface receptor. Membrane-bound immunoglobulin is non-signalling. It associates with two Ig-α/Ig-β heterodimers (members of the immunoglobulin gene superfamily), which have long cytoplasmic domains capable of transducing a signal.

The major histocompatibility complex (MHC)

HINTS AND TIPS

Major histocompatibility complex (MHC) is a generic term for a group of molecules produced by higher vertebrate species. The human leucocyte antigen (HLA) system is the human MHC.

The MHC genes

HINTS AND TIPS

A complete set of major histocompatibility complex (MHC) alleles inherited from one parent is referred to as a haplotype, and is found on the short arm of chromosome 6.

MHC genes exhibit a high degree of polymorphism, i.e. they exhibit considerable diversity (there are more than 100 identified alleles for human leucocyte antigen B (HLA-B)). This means that most individuals will be heterozygous at most MHC loci and that any two randomly selected individuals are very unlikely to have identical HLA alleles. Diversity of the MHC increases the chance that a person will be able to mount an adaptive response against a pathogen. The genetic loci are tightly linked, so that one set is inherited from each parent. The genes are divided into three regions, each region encoding one of the three classes of the MHC: class I, class II and class III (Fig. 10.3). The MHC alleles exhibit codominance, which means that both alleles are expressed.

Structure and function of the MHC

Class I and class II MHC molecules are glycoproteins expressed on the cell surface and consist of cytoplasmic, transmembrane and extracellular portions (Fig. 10.4).

Both class I and class II molecules exhibit broad specificity in their binding of peptide. The polymorphism of the MHC is largely concentrated in the peptide binding cleft.

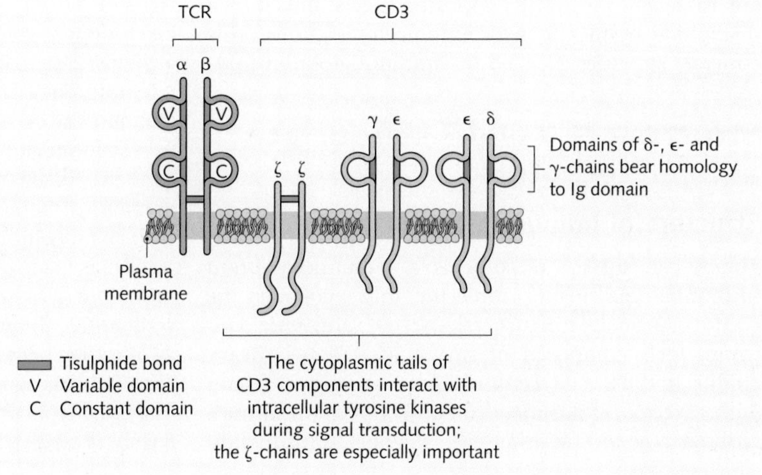

Fig. 10.2 Structure of the T cell surface antigen receptor. Negative charges on the transmembrane portion of CD3 components interact with positive charges on the T cell receptor (TCR). This maintains the complex. Antigen is detected by the TCR, but the signal is transduced by CD3.

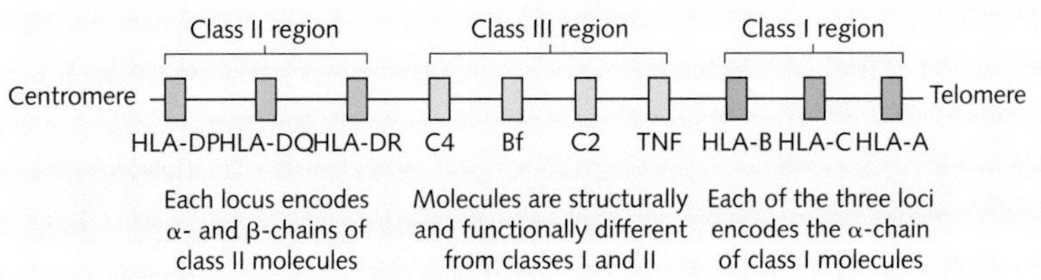

Fig. 10.3 Genetic organization of the human leucocyte antigen (HLA) complex. Only the classical genes are shown. The HLA complex is located in a 3–4 megabase sequence on the short arm of chromosome 6.

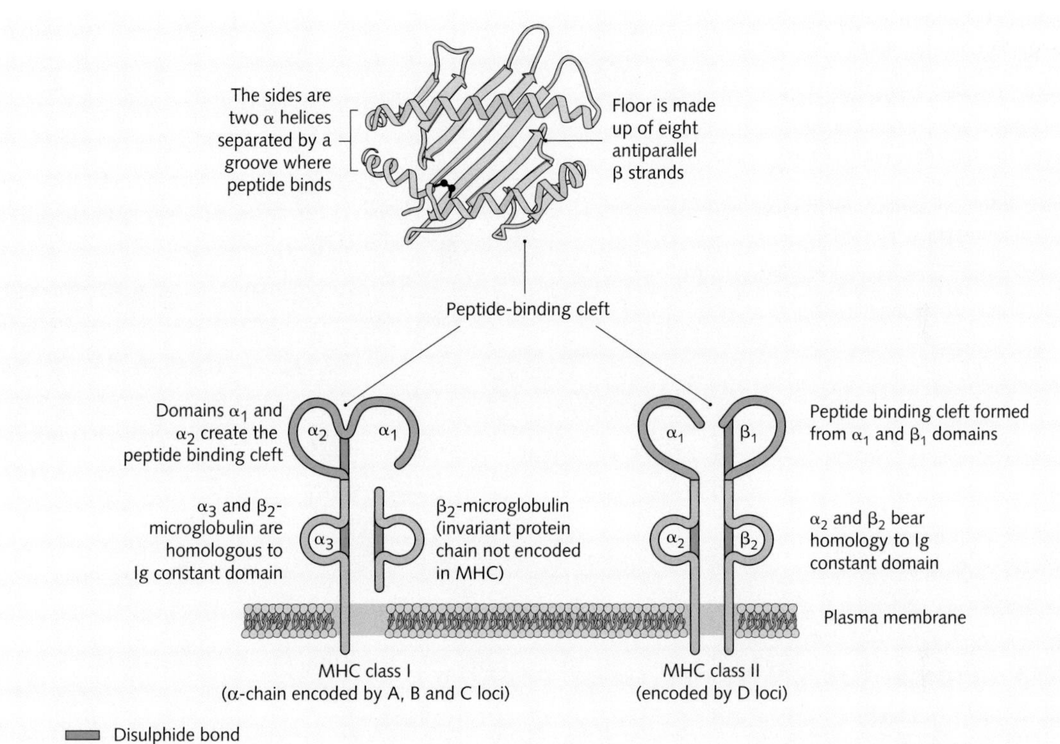

Fig. 10.4 Structure of class I and class II major histocompatibility molecules (MHC). The peptide binding cleft of a class I molecule is also shown as seen from above.

MHC restriction

T cells are only able to recognize antigen in the context of self-MHC molecules (self-MHC restriction). $CD8^+$ T cells recognize antigen only in association with class I MHC molecules (class I MHC restricted). $CD4^+$ cells recognize antigen only in association with class II MHC molecules (class II MHC restricted).

Antigen processing and presentation

MHC molecules do not present whole antigen, the antigen being degraded into peptide fragments before binding can occur. There are different pathways of antigen processing for class I and class II MHC; these pathways are summarized in Figure 10.5. Class I molecules are found on nearly all nucleated cells. Class I MHC molecules present endogenous antigens, such as those found in cells infected by viruses or intracellular bacteria. Thus $CD8^+$ T cells recognize virally altered cells and destroy them (see p. 112). Class II MHC molecules present exogenous antigens that may have been phago- or endocytosed into intracellular vesicles.

Professional antigen-processing cells process and present antigen to $CD4^+$ T cells in association with class II molecules. These cells express high levels of class II MHC molecules. Professional APCs include:

- Dendritic cells, including Langerhans' cells
- Macrophages
- B cells.

A summary of the differences between class I and class II MHC molecules is shown in Figure 10.6.

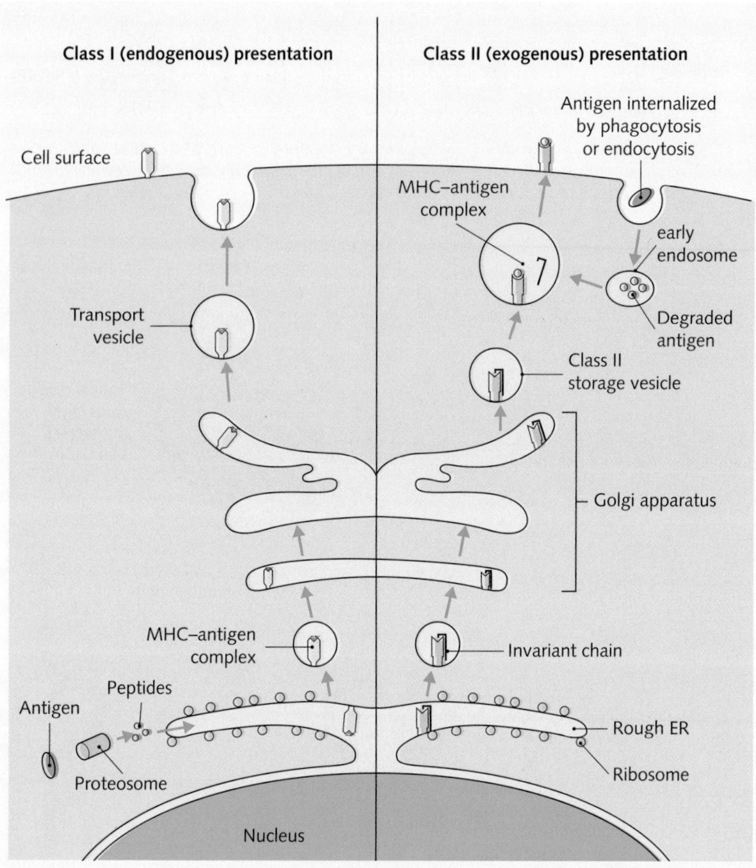

Fig. 10.5 Routes of antigen processing. Class I molecules present endogenous antigens. Cytosolic antigen is degraded by proteosomes and transported into the rough endoplasmic reticulum (ER), where peptides are loaded onto class I molecules. The MHC–peptide complex is transported via the Golgi apparatus to the cell surface. Class II molecules present exogenous antigens that have been phago- or endocytosed into intracellular vesicles. The MHC molecule is transported from the rough ER to the vesicle by the invariant chain (Ii). It is displaced from the MHC molecule by processed antigen, which is then presented at the cell surface. MHC, major histocompatibility complex.

Fig. 10.6 Differences between class I and class II major histocompatibility molecules

	Class I	Class II
Size of bound peptide	8–9 amino acids	13–18 amino acids (binding cleft more open)
Peptide from	Cytosolic antigen	Intravesicular or extracellular antigen
Expressed by	All nucleated cells, especially T cells, B cells, macrophages, other antigen-presenting cells, neutrophils	B cells, macrophages, other antigen-presenting cells, epithelial cells of the thymus, activated T cells
Recognized by	$CD8^+$ T cells	$CD4^+$ T cells

Structure and function of CD4 and CD8

CD4 and CD8 are 'accessory' molecules that play an important role in the T cell–antigen interaction. CD4 and CD8 have two important functions:

- They bind MHC class II and class I molecules, respectively, thereby strengthening the T cell–antigen interaction
- They function as signal transducers.

The role of CD4 and CD8 in antigen–receptor binding is shown in Figure 10.7.

GENERATION OF ANTIGEN RECEPTOR DIVERSITY

There are approximately 20^8 possible antigens, each requiring a corresponding receptor. The human genome contains only 30,000 genes and so each receptor

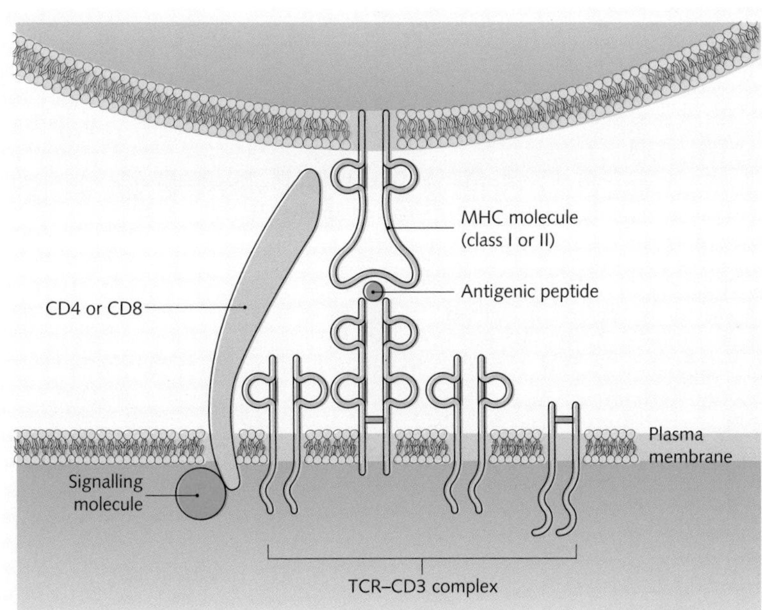

Fig. 10.7 The role of CD4 and CD8 in T cell receptor (TCR)-major histocompatibility complex (MHC) antigen interaction. CD4 or CD8 is closely associated with the TCR complex. They bind MHC in a restricted fashion (CD8 to class I only, CD4 to class II only). Binding is antigen independent and strengthens the bond between TCR and a complementary peptide-MHC complex. Molecules associated with CD4 or CD8 are then able to transduce a signal.

cannot be coded by a single gene. Instead this diversity is achieved by genetic recombination, a process where segments of information are cut and pasted from the gene.

T cell receptor and immunoglobulin are the only genes to undergo genetic recombination.

HINTS AND TIPS

Rearrangement of gene segments allows antibodies with an immense variety of specificity to be produced from a relatively small amount of DNA.

Genetic rearrangements

Before genetic recombination occurs, we say the gene segments are in germline configuration. Rearrangement only occurs in the variable domain (those that code for the active site) as the other segments of the receptor remain constant. Each variable domain is encoded by a random combination of one of each of the V, D (heavy chain only) and J exons (nucleic acid sequences). Following genetic rearrangement, one exon remains which codes for a variable domain. The C exons encode the constant regions. Heavy-chain C gene segments are clusters of exons, each of which encodes either a domain or a hinge region of the constant region.

Following rearrangement, the clonal progeny of each B cell will produce Ig of a single specificity. Rearrangement is completed and functional Ig chains are produced before the B cell encounters antigen (Fig. 10.8).

The presence of multiple V, D (heavy chain only) and J gene segments, and the apparently random selection of these segments, generates considerable diversity, which can be calculated (Fig. 10.9).

A similar process occurs in T cells: α- and γ-chain variable domains have V and J segments; β- and δ-chains have V, D and J segments.

Junctional diversity

The formation of junctions between the various gene segments produces an opportunity for increased diversity, where nucleotides are added or subtracted at random to form the joining segments.

Junctional flexibility and N-nucleotide addition

When exons are spliced, there are slight variations in the position of segmental joining. In addition, up to 15 nucleotides can be added to the D–J and the V–DJ joints. This occurs only in heavy chains and is catalysed by terminal deoxynucleotidyl transferase (TdT).

Both junctional flexibility and N-nucleotide addition can disrupt the reading frame, leading to non-functional rearrangements. However, formation of productive rearrangements increases antibody diversity. The V–J, V–DJ and VD–J joints fall within the antigen-binding region of the variable domain. Therefore, diversity generated at these joints will impact on the antigen specificity of the Ig molecule.

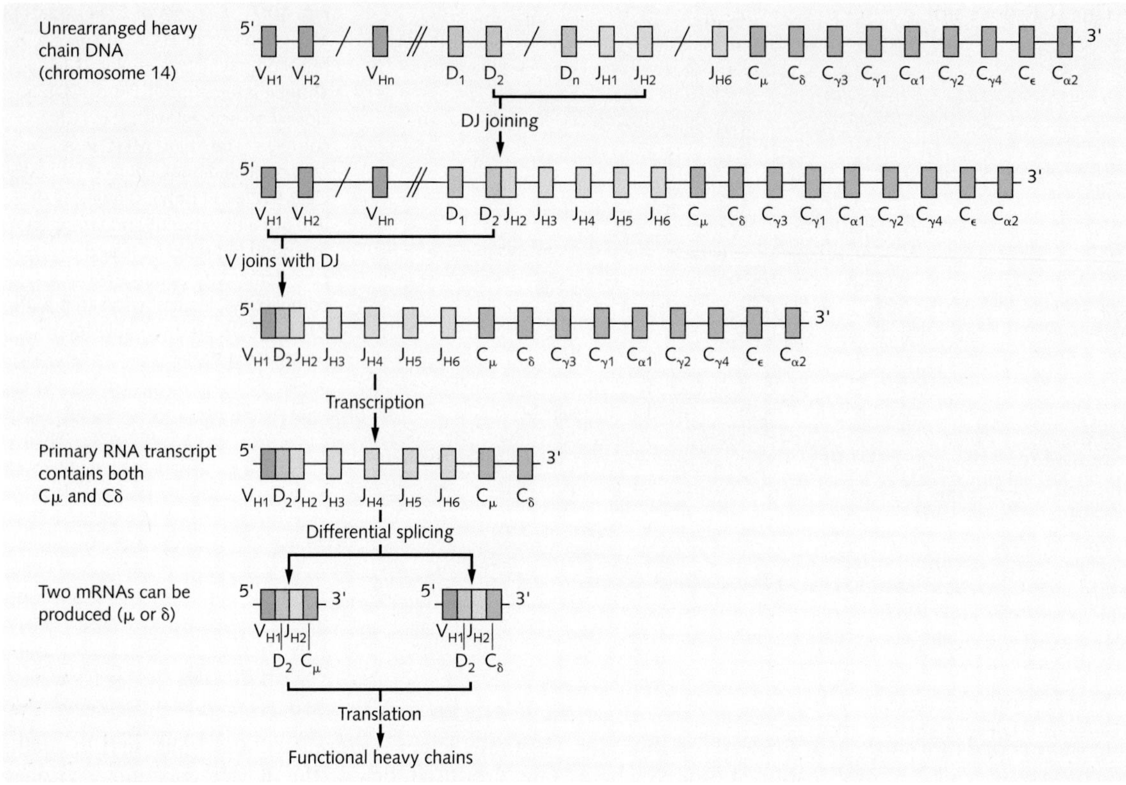

Fig. 10.8 Rearrangement of the heavy chain is similar to that of the light chain, although the join between D and J segments occurs first. In an unstimulated B cell, the heavy-chain mRNA that is transcribed contains both the Cμ and Cδ segments. The mRNA can be differentially spliced such that both IgM and IgD will be produced. They will both exhibit the same antigen binding specificity.

Fig. 10.9 Calculation of antibody diversity

Mechanism of diversity	**Number of combinations**		
	κ light chain	**λ light chain**	**Heavy chain**
Random joining of gene segments	$100 \times 5 = 500$	$100 \times 6 = 600$	$75 \times 30 \times 6 = 13{,}500$
Random chain associations	$(500 + 600) \times 13{,}500 = 1.5 \times 10^7$		

Given the fact that light chain can associate with any heavy chain, and from the number of gene segments present in germline DNA, it is possible to calculate the number of different molecules that can be produced. The extent of the contribution of junctional flexibility, N-nucleotide addition and somatic hypermutation is not known but will be significant.

Somatic hypermutation

Somatic hypermutation is a process that increases the affinity of antibody for its antigen and is also called affinity maturation. B cells that are dividing by mitosis to increase in number in order to combat infection are allowed to undergo mutation in their variable domain (the only cells in the body permitted to do so). Some mutations decrease the antibody's specificity for the antigen and apoptosis is stimulated in these cells; others result in antibody of increased specificity—these are positively selected for. Antibodies produced later in the primary immune response, and in the secondary immune response, will therefore have an increased affinity for antigen.

The TCR does not exhibit somatic hypermutation. Diversity is generated only in developing T cells, which can be deleted if they are either self-reactive or non-functional.

Class switching

This is the process whereby a single B cell can produce different classes of Ig that have the same specificity. The mechanism is not well understood but involves 'switch sites'—DNA sequences located upstream from each heavy chain C gene segment (except C_δ). Possible mechanisms include:

- Differential splicing of the primary transcript (see Fig. 10.8)
- A looping out and deletion of intervening heavy chain C gene segments (and introns)
- Exchange of C gene segments between chromosomes.

This process underlies the class switch from IgM in the primary response to IgG, IgA or IgE in the secondary response. Cytokines are important in controlling the switch.

Recognition molecules and their diversity are important for the generation of a specific, adaptive immune response. The adaptive immune response can be humoral or cell-mediated.

HUMORAL IMMUNITY

B cells and antibody production

The humoral immune response is brought about by antibodies, which are particularly efficient at eliminating extracellular pathogens. Antigen can be cleared from the host by a variety of effector mechanisms, which are dependent on antibody class or isotype (see p. 99):

- Activation of complement, leading to lysis or opsonization of the microorganism
- Antibody-dependent cell-mediated cytotoxicity (ADCC)
- Neutralization of bacterial toxins and viruses
- Mucosal immunity (IgA-mediated)
- Degranulation of mast cells – (IgE and IgG mediated).

Activated and differentiated B cells, known as plasma cells, produce antibodies. An overview of B cell activation is given in Figure 10.10.

B cells are activated within follicles found in secondary lymphoid structures, e.g. lymph nodes and spleen, only if they encounter specific antigen. During proliferation, variable regions of the immunoglobulin genes undergo somatic hypermutation. This process occurs in the germinal centre of the follicle. Follicular dendritic cells present antigen, to which the B cells with the highest affinity will bind. This causes the expression of bcl-2, which prevents B cells undergoing apoptosis. Therefore, the highest-affinity clones are positively selected. In order for B cells to produce antibody, they require help from T cells. Activated T helper cells provide the help needed by producing cytokines (IL-2, IL-4, IL-5, and IL-6). This acts as a further method of regulation within the immune system, as both B cells and T cells need exposure to the offending antigen in order for a response to be evoked. An overview of clonal selection of B cells is given in Figure 10.11.

Structure and function of antibody

The structure of immunoglobulin is shown in Figure 10.12.

Immunoglobulin molecules (using IgG as an example) are composed of two identical heavy and two identical light chains, linked by disulphide bridges. The light chains consist of one variable and one constant domain, while the heavy chain contains one variable and three constant domains. Digestion of IgG with papain (papaya protinase 1, an enzyme derived from papayas) produces two types of fragment:

1. Two Fab fragments (bind antigen) consisting of the light chain and two domains of the heavy chain (denoted VH and CH1)
2. One Fc fragment (binds complement) consisting of the remainder of the heavy chain (CH2 and CH3).

The light chain

The light chain is comprised of a variable, amino (N) terminal domain and a constant domain at the carboxy (C) terminal.

The constant region can be κ or λ, but both light chains within an Ig molecule will be the same; ≈60% of human light chains are κ.

The heavy chain

The heavy chain has a variable domain attached to several constant domains. There are five classes of immunoglobulin (Ig) in humans: IgG, IgA, IgM, IgE and IgD. The heavy chain determines the immunoglobulin class. The heavy chain can be γ (IgG), α (IgA), μ (IgM), ε (IgE) or δ (IgD). IgG, IgA and IgD have three constant domains with a hinge region; IgM and IgE have four constant domains but no hinge region.

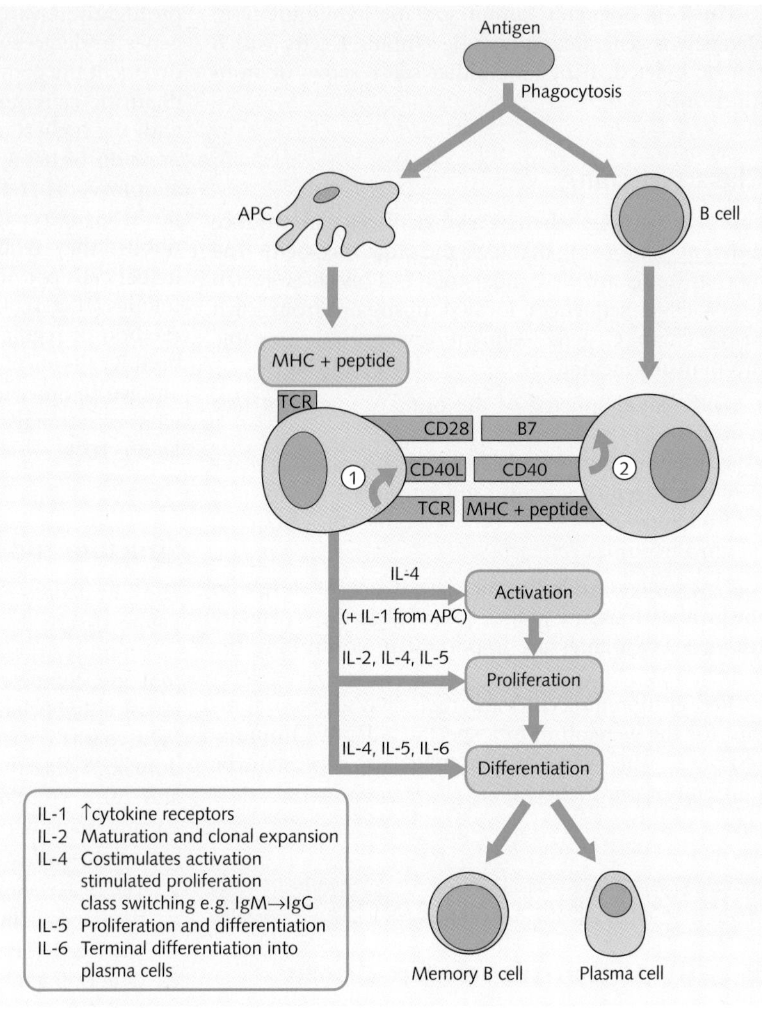

Fig. 10.10 Overview of the humoral immune response. Activated and differentiated B cells, known as plasma cells, produce antibody. B cells are activated by antigen in a T-cell-independent or dependent fashion. T helper cells are primed by antigen-presenting cells (APCs), which present antigen in conjunction with MHC class II molecules. B cells are stimulated by antigen interacting with B cell receptors. Primed T helper cells interact with B cells that also express antigen–MHC complexes. This interaction induces a sequence of surface receptor binding and cytokine production that results in B-cell activation, proliferation and differentiation. (1) Binding of the T cell receptor (TCR) to MHC induces the T cell to produce CD40L, which binds to CD40 on the B cell, producing a major stimulatory signal. (2) CD28 on the T cell then interacts with B7 on the B cell (costimulatory signal). Cytokines are also involved; their actions are shown in the diagram.

The variable domain

Each variable domain exhibits three regions that are hypervariable. The hypervariable regions on both light and heavy chains are closely aligned in the immunoglobulin molecule. Together, they form the antigen-binding site and therefore determine the molecule's specificity.

The hinge region

The hinge allows movement and therefore greater interaction with epitopes. The hinge region is also the site of the interchain disulphide bonds.

Classes of antibody

The different properties of the immunoglobulin classes are shown in Figure 10.13. Different Ig classes and subclasses are specific to each species. IgG, IgE and IgD are monomeric, secreted IgA (sIgA) is usually present as a dimer, and secreted IgM as a pentamer. The sIgA molecule is made up of two IgA monomers: a J chain and a secretory piece. The IgA dimer (J chain) is produced by submucosal plasma cells and enters the mucosal epithelial cell via receptor-mediated endocytosis, binding to the poly-Ig receptor. Having passed from the basal to the luminal surface of the epithelial cell, the IgA dimer is secreted across the mucosa, with part of the poly-Ig receptor (the secretory piece) still attached.

The functions of antibodies

The functions of Igs are shown in Figure 10.14.

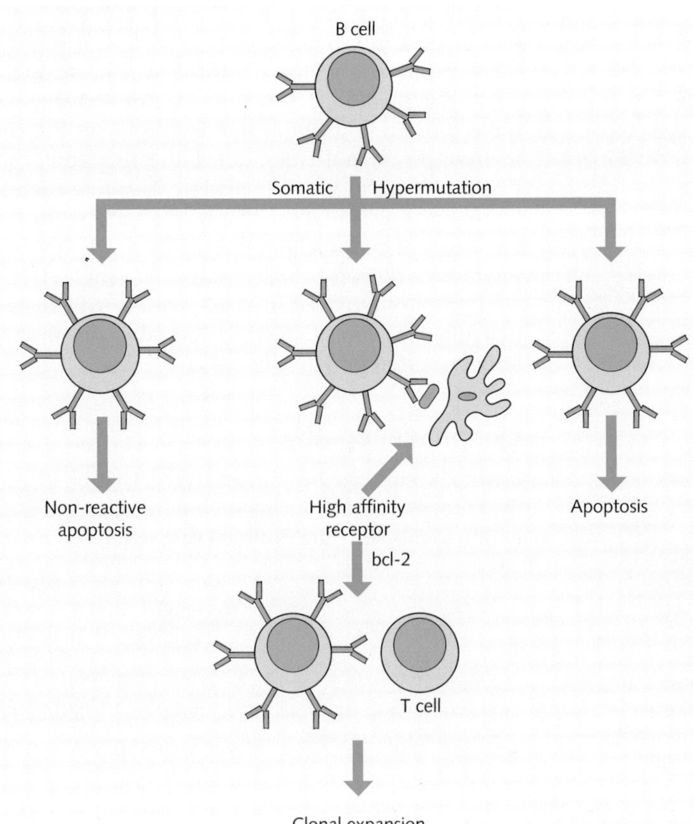

Fig. 10.11 Clonal selection of B cells. During B cell activation, the antigen-binding region of the immunoglobulin gene undergoes hypermutation. Clonal selection ensures that cells that produce the best antibody are selected and that non-functional or self-reactive B cells are deleted. This process occurs within the germinal centres of lymphoid follicles.

Lymphatic drainage and lymph nodes

Lymph nodes are secondary lymphoid organs. They provide a site for lymphocytes to interact with antigen and other cells of the immune system.

At the arterial end of capillaries, water and low-molecular-weight solutes are forced out into tissue spaces due to high hydrostatic pressure, creating interstitial fluid. Most interstitial fluid returns to the venous circulation at the venous end of capillaries (due to osmotic pressure gradients). The remainder leaves the interstitial space via the lymphatic system. Once interstitial fluid has entered a lymphatic vessel it is known as lymph. Lymphatic vessels are present in almost all tissues and organs of the body.

Lymphatic circulation

The lymphatic system acts as a passive drainage system to return interstitial fluid to the systemic circulation; lymph is not pumped around the body. Lymph vessels therefore contain numerous valves to prevent backflow of lymph. Afferent lymph vessels carry lymph into lymph nodes. They empty into the subcapsular sinus and lymph percolates through the node. Each node is drained by only one efferent vessel.

Lymph returns to the circulation at lymphovenous junctions. These are located at the junction of the right subclavian vein and right internal jugular vein (which empties the right lymphatic duct) and at the junction of the left subclavian vein and left internal jugular vein (which empties the thoracic duct).

Lymph nodes

Lymph nodes act as filters, 'sampling' lymphatic fluid for bacteria, viruses and foreign particles. APCs, loaded with antigen, also migrate through lymph nodes. They are present throughout the lymphatic system, often occurring at junctions of the lymphatic vessels. Lymph nodes frequently form chains, and may drain a specific organ or area of the body.

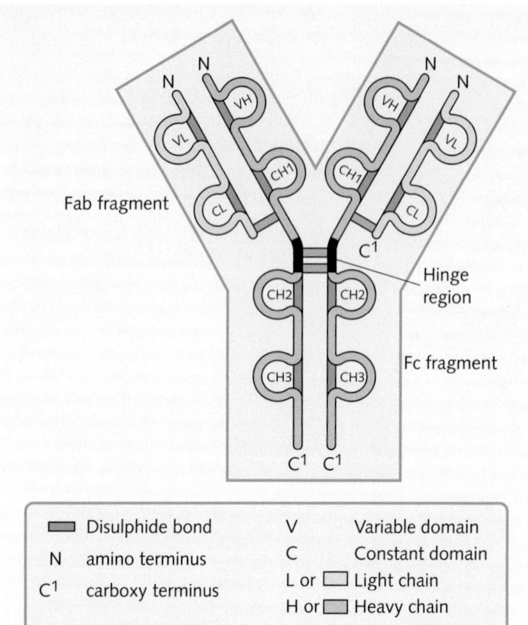

Fig. 10.12 Structure of IgG. Immunoglobulins are composed from two identical light and two identical heavy chains. The chains are divided into domains, each of which is an immunoglobulin fold. The variable domains form the antigen-binding site. Digestion of the immunoglobulin molecule with papain produces an Fc portion (which binds complement) and two Fab portions (which bind antigen).

Lymph nodes act as sites for initiation of the adaptive immune response. Antigen is sampled, processed and presented by several professional APCs (macrophages and dendritic cells).

Lymphocyte recirculation

Lymphocytes move continuously between blood and lymph. Efferent lymph contains more lymphocytes than afferent lymph because:

- Antigenic challenge results in stimulation and proliferation of lymphocytes
- Lymphocytes enter the lymph node directly from blood.

Lymphocyte recirculation is essential for a normal immune response (Fig. 10.15). Approximately 1–2% of the lymphocytic pool recirculates each hour. This increases the chances of an antigenically committed lymphocyte encountering complementary antigen.

Lymphocytes tend to recirculate to similar tissues. For example, an activated lymphocyte that has migrated from the skin to a local lymph node is most likely to migrate back to the skin following transport in the blood. Similarly, lymphocytes activated in mucosal-associated lymphoid tissue (MALT) will return to MALT. This recirculation is governed by the expression of molecules on both the lymphocyte and surface endothelium. These molecules, called integrins, confer specificity to lymphocyte recirculation. This fine tuning of lymphocyte recirculation is known as lymphocyte homing. Areas of endothelium through which lymphocytes migrate are known as high endothelial venules (HEVs). Lymphocytes activated in MALT express $\alpha_4\beta_7$ integrins that interact with MadCAM-1, an adhesion molecule only expressed on HEVs in MALT.

Lymphadenopathy

Lymph nodes can become enlarged (lymphadenopathy) for several reasons, including infection. Causes of lymphadenopathy are outlined on page 7.

HINTS AND TIPS

Lymphadenopathy can be a sign of infection. Understanding the drainage of lymph can lead you to the source of infection.

Mucosal-associated lymphoid tissue (MALT)

MALT consists of unencapsulated subepithelial lymphoid tissue found in the gastrointestinal, respiratory and urogenital tracts (Fig. 10.16).

It can be subdivided into:

- Organized lymphoid tissue, e.g. tonsils, appendix, Peyer's patches
- Diffuse lymphoid tissue located in the lamina propria of intestinal villi and lungs.

Organized lymphoid tissue

Respiratory tract

MALT in the nose and bronchi includes the:

- Lingual, palatine and nasopharyngeal tonsils
- Adenoids
- Bronchial nodules.

The respiratory system is exposed to a large number of organisms every day, most of which are cleared by the mucociliary escalator. Microorganisms that are not removed are presented by dendritic cells in the bronchi and stimulate germinating centres.

Fig. 10.13 Properties of the five immunoglobulin (Ig) classes

	IgG	IgA	IgM	IgE	IgD
Physical properties					
Molecular weight (kDa)	150	300	900	190	150
Serum concentration (mg/mL)	13.5	3.5	1.5	0.0003	0.03
Number of subunits	1	2	5	1	1
Heavy chain	γ	A	μ	ε	δ
Subclasses	4	2	—	—	—
Biological activities					
Present in secretions	✗	✓	✓	✗	✗
Crosses placenta	✓	✗	✗	✗	✗
Complement fixation	✓	✓	✓✓✓	✗	✗
Binds phagocytic receptors	✓	✗	✓	✗	✗
Binds mast cell receptors	✓	✗	✗	✓	✗
Other features					
Main role	Main circulatory Ig for secondary immune response	Major Ig in secretions	Main Ig in primary immune response	Allergy and antiparasitic response	Expressed on naïve B cell; function not known

Fig. 10.14 Summary of the functions of immunoglobulins

Function	Notes
Opsonization	Phagocytic cells have antibody (Fc) receptors, thus antibody can facilitate phagocytosis of antigen
Agglutination	Antigen and antibody (IgG or IgM) clump together because immunoglobulin can bind more than one epitope simultaneously. IgM is more efficient because it has a high valency (10 antigen-binding sites)
Neutralization	Binding to pathogens or their toxins prevents their attachment to cells
Antibody-dependent cell-mediated cytotoxicity (ADCC)	The antibody–antigen complex can bind to cytotoxic cells (e.g. cytotoxic T cells, NK cells) via the Fc component of the antibody, thus targeting the antigen for destruction
Complement activation	IgG and IgM can activate the classical pathway; IgA can activate the alternative pathway
Mast cell degranulation	Cross-linkage of IgE bound to mast cells and basophils results in degranulation
Protection of the neonate	Transplacental passage of IgG and the secretion of sIgA in breast milk protect the newborn

sIgA, secretory immunoglobulin A; NK, natural killer.

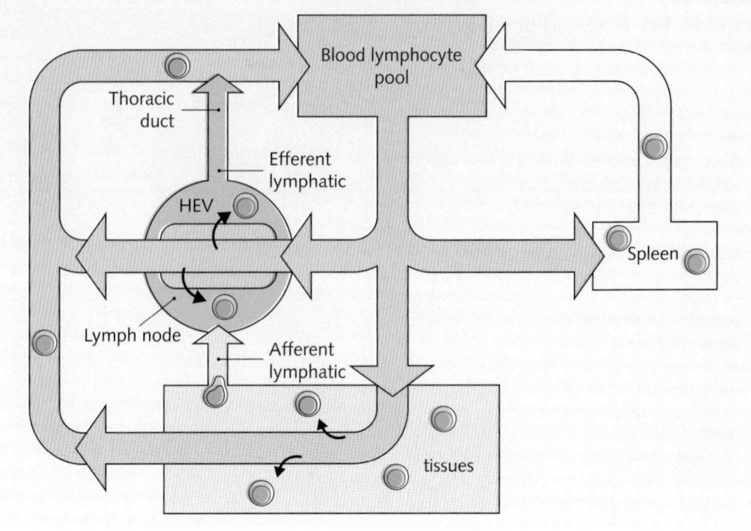

Fig. 10.15 Lymphocyte recirculation. Lymphocytes can enter lymph nodes via specialized high endothelial venules or in lymph. They leave the node in lymph that is returned to the systemic circulation via the right lymphatic duct or thoracic duct. HEV, high endothelial venule.

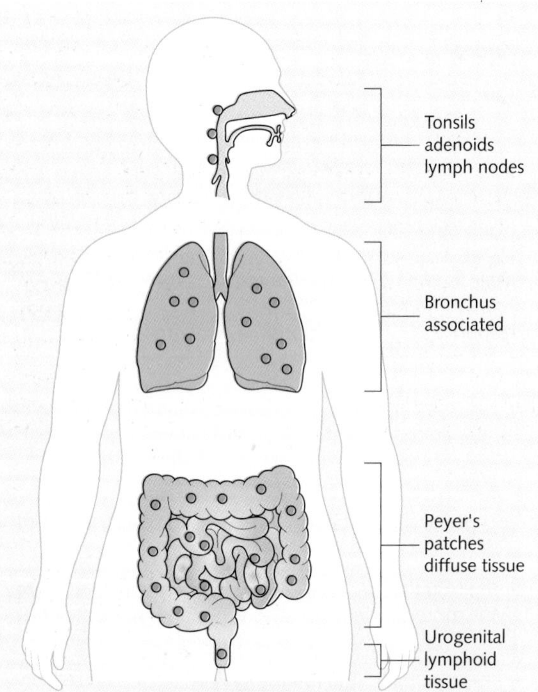

Fig. 10.16 Anatomical location of mucosal-associated lymphoid tissue (MALT). MALT is found in the nasal cavity, throat, respiratory tract, gastrointestinal tract and urogenital tract. Immune cells activated in MALT will home only to other mucosal sites.

Gastrointestinal tract

Peyer's patches are organized submucosal lymphoid follicles present throughout the large and small intestine, being particularly prominent in the terminal ileum. The structure of a Peyer's patch is shown in Figure 10.17.

Lymphocyte trafficking in MALT

Mucosal lymphocytes generally recirculate within the mucosal lymphoid system. This occurs through recognition between specific adhesion molecules on the surfaces of lymphocytes from Peyer's patches and corresponding ligands on the venular endothelium.

CELL-MEDIATED IMMUNITY

Cell-mediated immunity is mediated by T lymphocytes, macrophages and NK cells. The cell-mediated immune system is involved in the elimination of:

- Intracellular pathogens and infected cells (mainly viruses, mycobacteria and fungi)
- Tumour cells
- Foreign grafts.

The thymus plays an important role in cell-mediated immunity because it is the site of T cell maturation.

The thymus gland

The thymus is important for the production of T lymphocytes, selection of those which will recognize self-MHC and deletion of those that recognize self-antigen. T lymphocyte differentiation begins in the bone marrow (see p. 2) before early precursor cells migrate to the thymus. In the thymus, immature T lymphocytes undergo random recombination of their T cell receptor genes. Some of the resulting T cell receptors will be specific for pathogens and others for normal self-antigens. The role of the thymus is to select for cells that

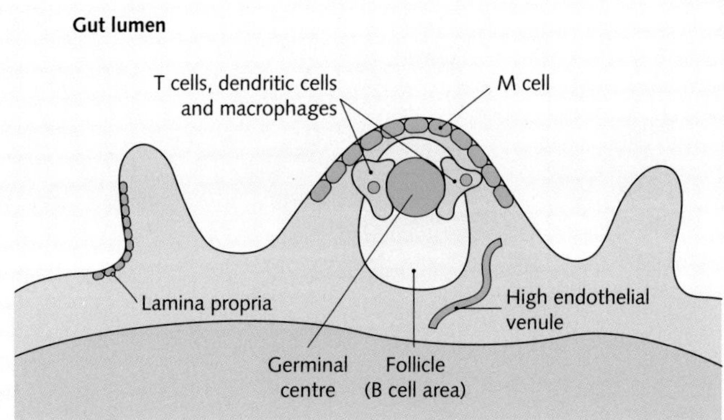

Fig. 10.17 Structure of a Peyer's patch. Peyer's patches are found in the gastrointestinal tract. Microbes are transported across specialized epithelial M cells in pinocytotic vesicles into a dome-shaped area. Antigen-presenting cells then process and present antigen to T cells. T helper cells can then activate B cells within the follicle. Some of the B cells do not differentiate into plasma cells, but migrate into germinal centres where they undergo high affinity and class switching maturation.

recognize self-MHC, and negatively select those T cells that recognize self-antigen with self-MHC.

The thymus is a gland with two lobes, located in the anterior part of the superior mediastinum, posterior to the sternum and anterior to the great vessels and upper part of the heart. It can extend superiorly into the root of the neck and inferiorly into the anterior mediastinum. It receives its blood supply from the inferior thyroid and internal thoracic arteries. Each lobe is surrounded by a capsule and is divided into multiple lobules by fibrous septa known as trabeculae. Each lobule is divided into two regions (Fig. 10.18):

- An outer cortex
- An inner medulla.

Immature thymocytes (T cell progenitors) enter the thymus gland via the cortex, where they rapidly proliferate and rearrange their T cell receptor genes. They then migrate towards the medulla where they encounter specialized epithelial cells. These cells express MHC class I and class II molecules. T cells that are able to bind self-MHC to some extent will proliferate, resulting in positive selection. The thymic epithelial cells have a unique mechanism for expressing many of the body's proteins (e.g. insulin) and peptides from these proteins are displayed on MHC class I and class II molecules. T cells which recognize this self-antigen can be forced to undergo apoptosis—so-called negative selection. A much smaller and more mature group of thymocytes survives to enter the medulla. Thymocytes continue to mature in the medulla and eventually leave the thymus, via post-capillary venules, as mature, antigen-specific, immunocompetent T cells. In total, only 1–5% of thymocytes in the thymus reach maturity, the remainder undergoing programmed cell death (apoptosis). The T cells which

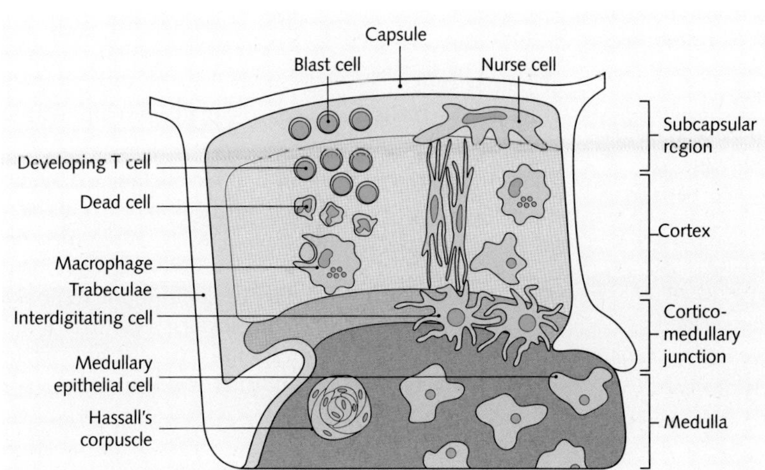

Fig. 10.18 Structure of a thymic lobule. The thymus is a bilobed gland, surrounded by a collagenous capsule, which is subdivided into lobules. Developing T cells (thymocytes) move from the subcapsular region to the medulla during maturation. Several different types of stromal cell support them. Many thymocytes undergo apoptosis (particularly in the cortex) and are phagocytosed by macrophages.

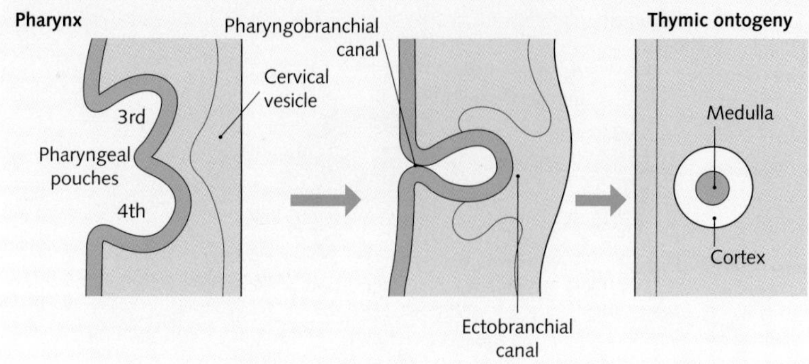

Fig. 10.19 Embryological development of the thymus. The thymus develops from the third (and possibly fourth) pharyngeal pouch. This forms the medulla, which is surrounded by the ectobranchial canal formed from the cervical vesicle. The thymus is developed by 8 weeks of gestation.

leave the thymus have been selected because they can recognize self-MHC, but those that recognize self-MHC plus antigen have been deleted.

Embryological origin of the thymus

The human embryonic thymus develops from the third pharyngeal pouch during week 4 or 5 of gestation (Fig. 10.19).

The thymus gland is formed by week 8, and is fully differentiated and producing viable lymphocytes by week 17. The third pharyngeal pouch also gives rise to the parathyroid glands. Lymphoid stem cells are produced by the fetal liver and spleen, and by bone marrow from 6 months' gestation.

Thymic hypoplasia

Although it continues to grow until puberty, the relative size of the thymus gland decreases over this period. After puberty there is a real reduction in size and, by adulthood, it is composed largely of adipose tissue and produces far fewer T lymphocytes. This means it is harder for adults to recover from immunological damage caused by, for example, HIV or immunosuppressive drugs.

DiGeorge syndrome is an autosomal dominant condition, caused by a deletion on chromosome 22 (22q11.2). Defects in the third and fourth pharyngeal pouch can result in thymic aplasia, heart defects, hypoparathyroidism and cleft palate, among other anomalies. Thymic aplasia leads to an absence of circulating T cells and a reduction in cell-mediated immunity. The mother provides no passive T cell immunity after birth and infants present early with infections.

T lymphocytes

Functions of different T cell phenotypes

The different types of T cell can be differentiated by cell-surface molecules and function. There are two different types of T cell receptor (TCR), which have different functions. T cells expressing $\alpha\beta$-TCRs account for at least 95% of circulatory T cells. They become cytotoxic, helper or suppressor cells and, unless specified otherwise, account for all the T cells mentioned in this book. T cells expressing a $\gamma\delta$-TCR are present at mucosal surfaces and their specificity is biased towards certain bacterial and viral antigens. Some $\gamma\delta$-T cells can recognize antigen independently of an APC. These T cells are usually cytotoxic in their actions. They differ from NK cells because they detect antigen rather than the presence or absence of MHC class I molecules. They are part of the adaptive system, because their action is specific and shows evidence of immunological memory.

T helper cells

T helper (Th) cells play a key role in the development of the immune response:

- They determine the epitopes that are targeted by the immune system via their interactions with antigen in conjunction with class II MHC molecules on APCs
- They determine the nature of the immune response directed against target antigens, e.g. cytotoxic T cell response or antibody response
- They are required for normal B cell function (see p. 97).

Fig. 10.20 Differences between the T helper 1 (Th1), T helper 2 (Th2) and T helper 17 (Th17) cell subsets

Cytokines secreted	**Th1 cells** ***IL-2, IFN-γ, TNF-β***	**Th2 cells** ***IL-4, IL-10***	**Th17 cells** ***IL-17***
Functions	• Responsible for classical cell-mediated immunity reactions such as delayed-type hypersensitivity and cytotoxic T cell activation • Involved in responses to intracellular pathogens, for example viruses, some protozoa and fungi and most bacteria • Activate macrophages	• Promote B cell activation • Involved in allergic diseases and responses to helminthic infections • Involved in responses to extracellular pathogens, mostly bacteria	• Promote neutrophil activation and migration • Involved in responses to bacteria and fungi

Most Th cells are $CD4^+$ and can be divided into five subsets on the basis of the cytokines they secrete:

1. Th0
2. Th1
3. Th2
4. Th17
5. Treg.

Th0 cells arise as a result of initial short-term stimulation of naïve T cells; they are capable of secreting a broad spectrum of cytokines. Prolonged stimulation results in the emergence of Th1 and Th2 subsets. The cytokines released by the Th1 and Th2 subsets modulate one another's secretion. The different cytokine profiles of the Th1, Th2 and Th17 subsets reflect their different immunological functions (Fig. 10.20).

Most immune responses involve more than one subset of T cells. For example staphylococcus (an extracellular bacterium) stimulates both Th2 and Th17 responses. On the other hand, some responses become very polarized. For example, the immune system relies almost exclusively on Th1 cells to respond to mycobacterium tuberculosis, an intracellular pathogen.

The fifth type of helper T cell has two main regulatory roles. The first is to dampen down the immune response once an infection has been brought under control. The second is to regulate self-reactive T cells which have managed to escape negative selection in the thymus. Their action is via cytokines, including transforming growth factor-β (TGF-β) and IL-10.

Cytotoxic T cells

Most cytotoxic T (Tc) lymphocytes are $CD8^+$ and recognize antigen in conjunction with class I MHC molecules (endogenous antigen). They lyse target cells via the same mechanisms as NK cells (see p. 84).

Development of T cells

T cell precursors are produced in the bone marrow and are transported to the thymus for development and maturation. The aim of T cell development and maturation is to select T cells with receptors that can recognize foreign antigens in conjunction with self-MHC. Cells with non-functioning receptors or that are strongly self-reactive are destroyed (Fig. 10.21).

Positive selection

Positive selection occurs in the thymic cortex. T cells that are capable of binding self-MHC are allowed to live, i.e. they are positively selected for, and T cells that do not recognize self-MHC die. Furthermore, T cells that interact with MHC class I lose their CD4 (they are now CD8 T cells) and T cells that interact with MHC class II lose their CD8 (becoming CD4 T cells); this is MHC restriction. T cells that do not interact with the MHC molecules undergo apoptosis, as they do not receive a protective signal as a result of the TCR–MHC interaction.

Negative selection

T cells that are positively selected, but have high affinity for MHC molecules and self-antigen, undergo negative selection. Because thymic epithelial cells express many different proteins from around the body, this mechanism destroys most self-reactive T cells.

T cell activation

T cells are activated by interactions between the TCR and peptide bound to MHC. Activation also requires a 'second message' from the antigen-presenting cell. This process is shown in Figure 10.22.

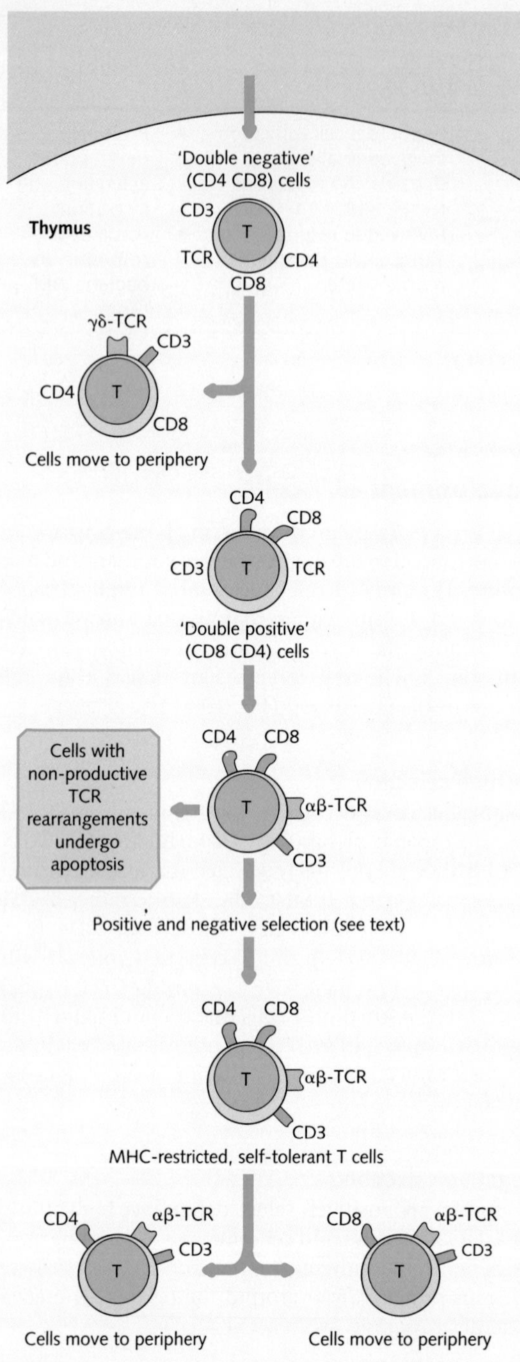

Fig. 10.21 Development of T cells in the thymus. Cells entering the thymus to become T cells are negative for CD4, CD8, CD3 and the T cell receptor (TCR). Rearrangement of the genes encoding the TCR will produce three cell lines: (1) $CD4^+$ αβ-TCR; (2) $CD8^+$ αβ-TCR; and (3) $CD4^-CD8^-$ γδ-TCR. The β- or γ-chain genes rearrange first. If a functional β-chain is formed, both CD4 and CD8 are upregulated and the α-chain gene rearranges. The resultant T cells are positively selected if their TCR is functional, but negatively selected if they react too strongly. The majority of thymocytes will undergo apoptosis due to positive or negative selection. MHC, major histocompatibility complex.

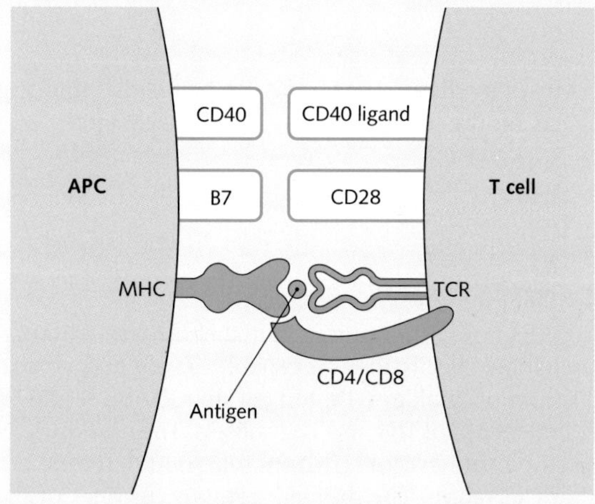

Fig. 10.22 Activation of T cells. Several interactions with antigen-presenting cells (APCs) are required to activate T cells. The T cell receptor (TCR) and CD4 or CD8 bind to MHC and antigen. CD28 on the T cell binds to B7 on the APC, providing a co-stimulatory signal. MHC, major histocompatibility complex.

Once T cells are activated they produce a wide range of molecules with several functions. These are primarily cytokines, which may be pro- or anti-inflammatory (see Fig. 10.20) or involved in activation of other immune cells.

Superantigens

T cells can be activated in a non-specific fashion by superantigens. Superantigens cross-link between the V-β domain of the TCR and a class II MHC molecule on an antigen-presenting cell. Cross-linking is independent of the peptide binding cleft but depends on the framework region of the V-β domain. This means that one superantigen is able to activate about 5% of T cells, far more than normal antigen. An example of a T cell superantigen is staphylococcal enterotoxin.

Superantigens result in polyclonal activation effectively 'crowding-out' the specific, protective immune response. A consequence of polyclonal activation can be autoimmune disease. Superantigen can also result in the deletion of a large number of T cells by inducing negative selection in the thymus.

Toxic shock syndrome (TSS)

Toxins produced by staphylococci and streptococci can act as superantigens, producing the clinical picture of 'toxic shock syndrome', where a seemingly innocuous stimulus such as a graze can lead to fever, a diffuse macular rash, hypotension and shock. There is an association between tampon use and *Staph. aureus* TSS, with many known deaths as a result. Management of TSS involves transfer to hospital, aggressive fluid resuscitation, as well as ventilatory and renal support. Antibiotic therapy should cover *Staph. aureus* and *Staph. pyogenes*.

The functioning immune system

Objectives

You should be able to:

- Outline the response of tissue to infection or injury
- Understand the molecular and physiological features of acute and chronic inflammation
- Explain the immune response to viruses, bacteria and protozoa.

RESPONSE TO TISSUE DAMAGE

Inflammation is a non-specific response evoked by tissue injury. The aims of the process are:

- Removal of the causative agent, e.g. microbes or toxins
- Removal of dead tissue
- Replacement of dead tissue with normal tissue, or scar formation.

HINTS AND TIPS

Inflammation is defined clinically by four cardinal signs: rubor, dolor, calor and tumor (redness, pain, heat and swelling). Histologically inflammation is defined by the presence of oedema and white cells in a tissue.

Acute inflammation

Acute inflammation is the immediate response to cell injury. It is of short duration (a few hours to a few days) and is triggered by a range of insults, including chemical or thermal damage and infection. Infection is sensed by resident macrophages, through Toll-like receptors, which then release cytokines, attracting neutrophils to the site of infection. In other instances, inflammation is initiated by resident mast cells, which tend to attract eosinophils. Once inflammation is initiated, several changes occur in vascular endothelium to allow attachment and extravasation of leucocytes—primarily neutrophils but also monocytes and lymphocytes. Attachment and extravasation require the presence of surface molecules on both the endothelium and leucocytes. The acute inflammation process is mediated by many different chemicals.

Vascular changes

Tissue injury results in the release of chemical mediators (cytokines, chemokines and histamine) that act on local blood vessels. The main changes that occur are:

- Vasodilatation: causing increased blood flow and therefore redness and heat
- Slowing of the circulation and increased vascular permeability: formation of an inflammatory exudate results in swelling
- Entry of inflammatory cells, especially neutrophils, into the tissues.

Leucocyte extravasation

Neutrophils adhere to the vessel wall and then pass between the endothelial cells into the tissues. This is a multistep process involving:

- Margination: adherence of neutrophils to the vessel wall. There are two phases to margination. The first is 'tethering and rolling' and the second is 'activation and strengthening'. Neutrophils adhere to vessel walls via cell adhesion molecules (CAMs). CAMs can be members of the immunoglobulin superfamily, the selectin family or the integrin family
- Diapedesis (extravasation): neutrophils move between endothelial cells into the tissue
- Chemotaxis: due to the release of several chemotactic agents (Fig. 11.1).

Integrin molecules allow immune cells to target specific sites (a process known as homing). To interact successfully with the extracellular matrix, neutrophils must express β_1-integrins, a set of adhesion molecules that can bind to collagen and laminin.

Once neutrophils reach a site of inflammation, they phagocytose foreign particles and release enzymes (see Chapter 9). Leucocytes can release proteases and metabolites during chemotaxis and phagocytosis, which are

Fig. 11.1 Overview of the mediators of acute inflammation

Action	Mediators
Increased vascular permeability	Histamine, bradykinin, C3a, C5a, leukotrienes C_4, D_4, E_4, PAF
Vasodilatation	Histamine, prostaglandins, PAF
Pain	Bradykinin, prostaglandins
Leucocyte adhesion	LTB_4, IL-1, TNF-α, C5a
Leucocyte chemotaxis	C5a, C3a, IL-8, PAF, LTB_4, fibrin and collagen fragments
Acute phase response	IL-1, TNF-α, IL-6
Tissue damage	Proteases and free radicals

IL, interleukin; LT, leukotriene; PAF, platelet-activating factor; TNF, tumour necrosis factor.

potentially harmful to the host. Neutrophils die during this process, creating pus.

Molecular mediators of inflammation

A variety of chemical mediators are produced during an inflammatory response. They usually have short half-lives and are rapidly inactivated by a variety of systems. A summary of their actions is given in Figure 11.1.

Cell membrane phospholipid metabolites

Prostaglandins (PGs) and leukotrienes (LTs) are derived from the metabolism of arachidonic acid. Platelet-activating factor (PAF) is also an important mediator.

Cytokines

Cytokines such as IL-8 and IL-1, and tumour necrosis factor-α (TNF-α) act to:

- Induce expression of CAMs on the endothelium, thus enhancing leucocyte adhesion
- Attract neutrophils to the area of injury
- Induce prostacyclin (PGI_2) production
- Induce PAF synthesis
- Mediate the development of the acute-phase response
- Stimulate fibroblast proliferation and increase collagen synthesis.

The complement system

This is discussed in Chapter 9.

The kinin system

Bradykinin is released following activation of the kinin system by clotting factor XII. Bradykinin increases vascular permeability and mediates pain.

The coagulation system

The coagulation system is activated at sites of vascular injury (see p. 63). Fibrinopeptides produced during coagulation are chemotactic for neutrophils and increase vascular permeability. Thrombin also promotes fibroblast proliferation and leucocyte adhesion.

The fibrinolytic system

Plasmin (see p. 65) has several functions in the inflammatory process, including:

- Activation of complement via C3
- Cleavage of fibrin to form 'fibrin degradation products', which may increase vascular permeability.

Results of acute inflammation

There are several possible outcomes resulting from acute inflammation. These include:

- Regrowth and resolution
- Healing by collagenous scar formation
- Abscess formation
- Chronic inflammation.

Chronic inflammation

Chronic inflammation arises:

- When the causative agent cannot be eliminated and antigenic persistence occurs. This may be due to deficiencies in the host response or certain microorganisms, e.g. *Mycobacterium tuberculosis*, which have evolved to evade the immune response
- As a result of persistent autoimmune reactions, e.g. systemic lupus erythematosus (SLE) and rheumatoid arthritis. The body is, of course, incapable of clearing autoantigens.

The key cells of chronic inflammation are macrophages, lymphocytes and plasma cells. This is in marked contrast to acute inflammation, which is characterized primarily by a neutrophilic inflammation. Ongoing inflammation is associated with tissue destruction, but also healing.

In chronic inflammation, macrophage numbers are increased because they are recruited by chemotactic factors (e.g. platelet-derived growth factor (PDGF) and C5a) and are prevented from leaving by migration inhibition factor. Macrophage secretory products mediate characteristic features of chronic inflammation:

- TNF probably has a key role in maintaining chronic inflammation at a local level. When it is secreted at high levels it has systemic effects, including weight loss (through fat catabolism and appetite inhibition) and fatigue
- Tissue damage via proteases and oxygen radicals
- Revascularization via angiogenic factors
- Fibroblast migration and proliferation via growth factors (e.g. PDGF) and cytokines (IL-2, TNF-α)

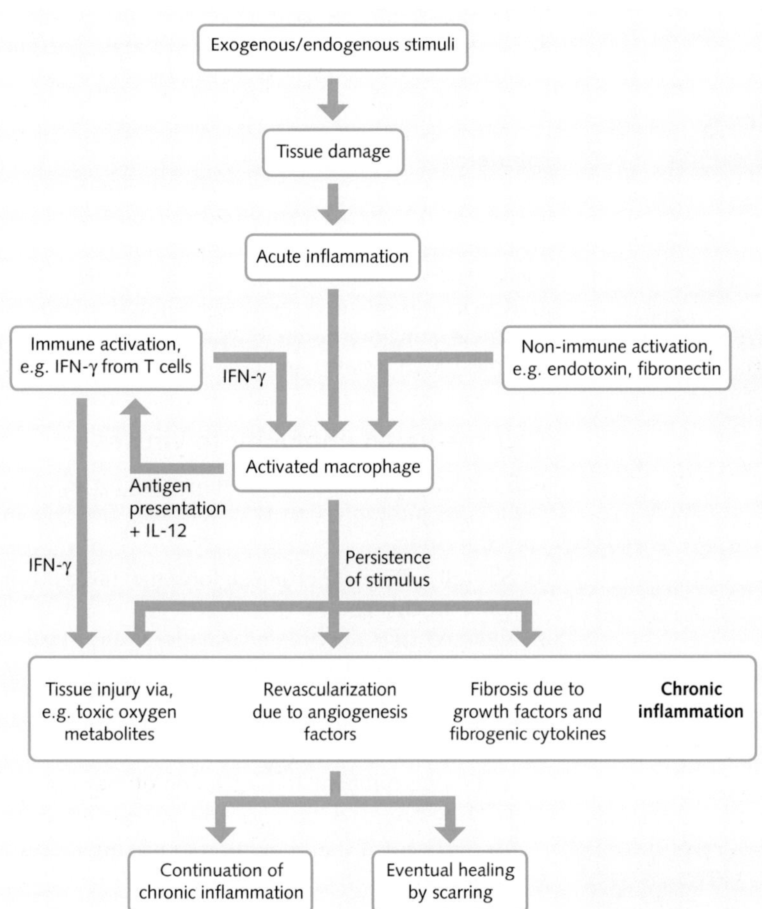

Fig. 11.2 Overview of chronic inflammation. Macrophages can be activated by T cells or by nonimmune mechanisms. Activated macrophages persist at sites of chronic inflammation because of persistent stimulation. They release a number of molecules, which produce the characteristic features of chronic inflammation. Macrophages act as antigen-presenting cells to T cells, which can then activate further macrophages.

- Collagen synthesis via growth factors (e.g. PDGF) and cytokines (IL-1, TNF-α)
- Remodelling via collagenases
- Simulation of T cell activity by secretion of IL-12.

Lymphocytes and plasma cells are also present at the site of inflammation. In the case of chronic infections, both macrophages and T cells are required to control infection. An overview of chronic inflammation is given in Figure 11.2.

Inflammation in disease

Inflammation is intended to protect the host but can, under certain circumstances, prove destructive. Antigenic persistence results in the continued activation and accumulation of macrophages. This leads to the formation of epithelioid cells (slightly modified macrophages) and granuloma formation (Fig. 11.3).

TNF-α is needed for granuloma formation and maintenance. Interferon-γ (IFN-γ), released by activated T cells, causes macrophage transformation into epithelioid and multinucleate giant cells (which arise from the fusion of several macrophages). The granuloma is surrounded by a cuff of lymphocytes and the migration of fibroblasts results in increased collagen synthesis. Caseous necrotic areas (dry, 'cheese-like' white mass of degenerated tissue) might be present in the centre of a granuloma.

The nature of the damaging stimulus determines the type of granuloma formed. Inert particles (e.g. silica in the lungs) are predominantly surrounded by macrophages. Microorganisms such as *M. tuberculosis* (which causes tuberculosis) induce a persistent, delayed-type hypersensitivity (DTH) response, resulting in granuloma formation in the lung and possibly leading to cavitation. The granuloma formed is characterized by focal accumulation of lymphocytes and macrophages. Phagocytosis of mycobacteria is not usually effective because the

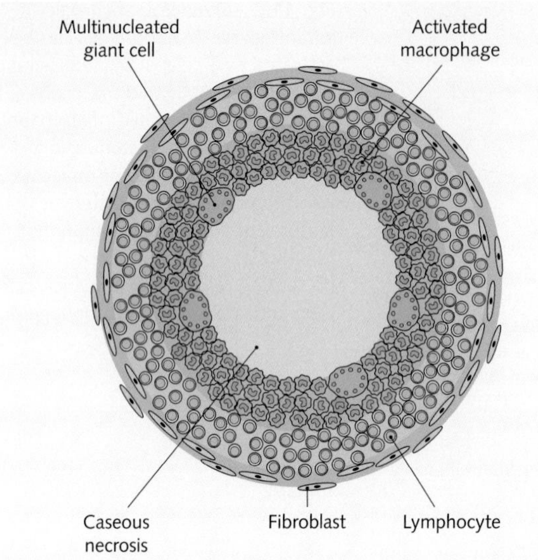

Fig. 11.3 A granuloma, showing typical focal accumulation of lymphocytes and macrophages around a central area of caseous necrosis.

microorganism can survive and multiply within macrophages. The granulomatous response, although preventing spread of infection, is harmful to the host.

IMMUNE RESPONSE TO PATHOGENS

Immune response to viral infection

Viruses do not always kill host cells but budding and release of new viral particles often causes the cells to lyse. The immune system can act to prevent infection or the spread of infection, or to eliminate an intracellular target once infection has occurred.

Humoral immunity to viruses

The humoral response is involved in preventing entry to, and viral replication within, cells.

Antibody

Antibodies can bind to free virus and prevent its attachment and entry to a cell; this is referred to as neutralization of virus particles (e.g. IgG neutralizes the hepatitis B virus on entering the blood stream and IgA neutralizes the influenza virus entering the nasal mucosa). Antibodies can also bind to viral proteins expressed on the surface of infected cells. Antibody bound to cells can initiate antibody-dependent cell-mediated cytotoxicity (ADCC) and complement activation, and acts as an opsonin for phagocytes.

Responses directed against free virus are considered to be the most important in vivo, and antibodies are, therefore, important early in the course of infection to prevent spread of virus between cells.

Interferon

Interferons (IFNs) are produced by virally infected cells. IFN-α and IFN-β act on neighbouring uninfected cells by inhibiting transcription and translation of viral proteins. IFN-γ activates macrophages and natural killer (NK) cells and enhances the adaptive immune response by upregulating expression of major histocompatibility complex (MHC) class I and class II molecules.

Cell-mediated immunity to viruses

Cell-mediated mechanisms are important for eliminating a virus once infection is established. The cells involved include:

- NK cells: these are cytotoxic for virus-infected cells and participate in ADCC
- Cytotoxic $CD8^+$ T cells: viral peptides are presented on the cell surface in association with class I MHC molecules. $CD8^+$ T cells can destroy these infected cells
- $CD4^+$ T cells: T helper cells are required for the generation of antibody and cytotoxic T cell responses, and the recruitment and activation of macrophages (Th1 help).

An overview of the immune response to viruses is given in Figure 11.4.

Examples of viral infection and strategies to avoid immunity

Viral infections are common and most are self-limiting. Some, particularly those that can evade the immune response, can be chronic and are potentially fatal (e.g. HIV [see p. 129] and hepatitis B). Different viruses use different strategies to evade the host's immune response:

- Antigenic shift and drift: these are mechanisms of antigenic variation, e.g. influenza
- Polymorphism: e.g. adenovirus, rhinovirus
- Latent virus: e.g. herpes simplex virus (HSV), varicella zoster
- Modulation of major histocompatibility complex (MHC) expression: cytomegalovirus (CMV), adenovirus, Epstein–Barr virus (EBV), HSV, HIV
- Infection of lymphocytes, e.g. HIV, measles, CMV, EBV.

Antigenic variation, either by mutation or polymorphism, circumvents immunological memory because the virus expresses different immunological targets over time. By becoming latent, a virus 'hides' from the immune system. A latent virus often reactivates when the immune system is compromised, suggesting that there must be some interaction between the immune system

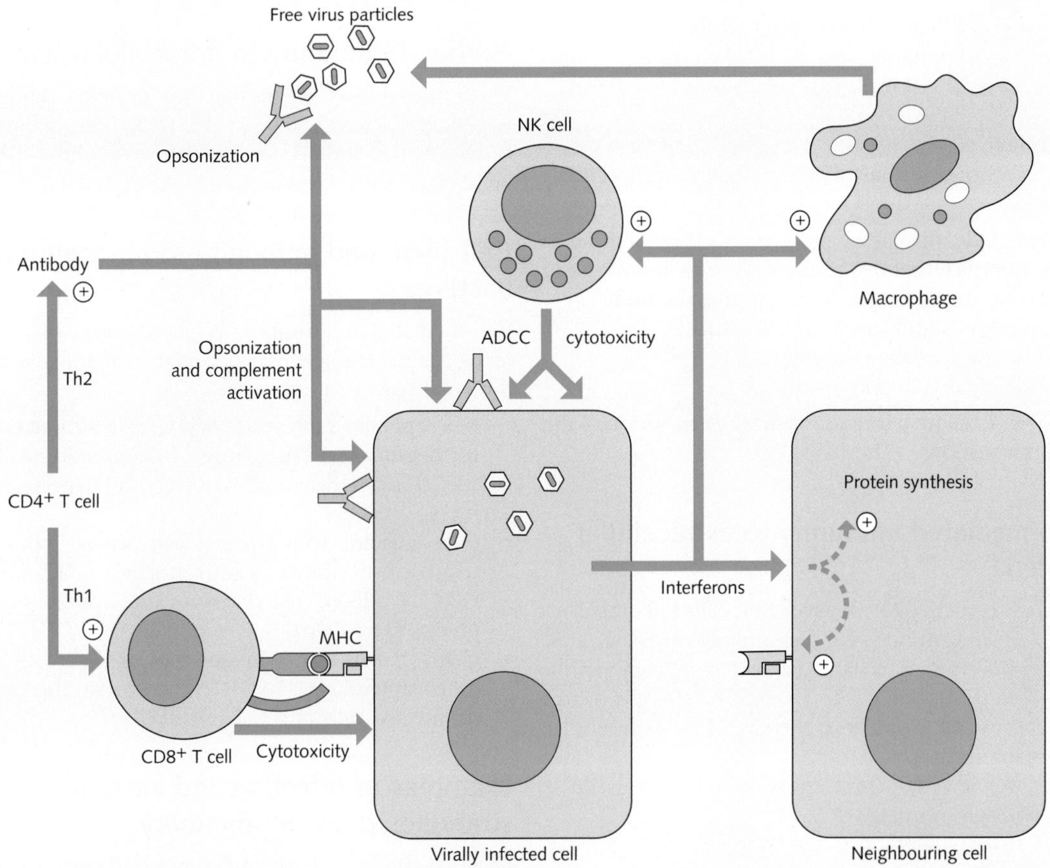

Fig. 11.4 The immune response to viruses. Interferons, produced by virally infected cells, have three important actions. Interferon-α and interferon-β induce an antiviral state in neighbouring cells (inhibition of viral transcription and translation). Interferon-γ activates macrophages and natural killer (NK) cells and upregulates major histocompatibility complex (MHC) molecules. NK cells kill virally infected cells either by detecting the absence of MHC class I molecules or by antibody-dependent cell-mediated cytotoxicity (ADCC). Macrophages phagocytose opsonized free virus and cell fragments, and produce further interferon. $CD8^+$ (cytotoxic) T cells sense viral peptides presented by MHC class I molecules and destroy the cell. $CD4^+$ (helper) T cells help to activate macrophages and are involved in the generation of antibody and cytotoxic T cell responses.

and the virus even when it is latent. Mechanisms that prevent normal effector functions from being carried out primarily involve down regulation of MHC class I expression. However, viruses can also interfere with IFN or produce inhibitory cytokines. Infection of lymphocytes, and their death, reduces the ability of the immune system to combat viral infection.

Immune response to bacterial infection

Bacteria are prokaryotic organisms. Their cell membrane is surrounded by a peptidoglycan cell wall. Many bacteria also have a capsule of large, branched polysaccharides. Bacteria attach to cells via surface pili, but only some bacteria enter host cells. Different immune mechanisms operate, depending on whether the bacteria are extracellular or intracellular.

Extracellular bacteria

Humoral immunity to extracellular bacteria

Complement

Bacteria activate complement via the lectin or alternative pathways. Activated complement products play a role in the elimination of bacteria, especially C3b (an opsonin), C3a and C5a (anaphylatoxins that recruit leucocytes), and the membrane attack complex (MAC), which can perforate the outer lipid bilayer of Gram-negative bacteria.

Lysozyme

Lysozyme is a naturally occurring antibacterial that attacks *N*-acetyl muramic acid–*N*-acetyl glucosamine links in the bacterial cell wall. This results in bacterial lysis.

Antibody

This is the principal defence against extracellular bacteria:

- sIgA binds to bacteria and prevents their binding to epithelial cells; if this response is sufficient, sIgA can prevent the pathogen from entering the body
- Antibody neutralizes bacterial toxins
- Antibody activates complement
- Antibody acts as an opsonin.

$CD4^+$ T cell help is required for the generation of the antibody response (Th2 help).

Cell-mediated immunity to extracellular bacteria

Phagocytic, particularly neutrophils, cells kill most bacteria; C3b and antibody enhance phagocytosis. Bacterial antigens are processed and presented in conjunction with class II MHC to $CD4^+$ T cells. Th17 T cells recruit and activate neutrophils to the site of an extracellular bacterial infection.

An overview of the immune response to extracellular bacteria is given in Fig. 11.5.

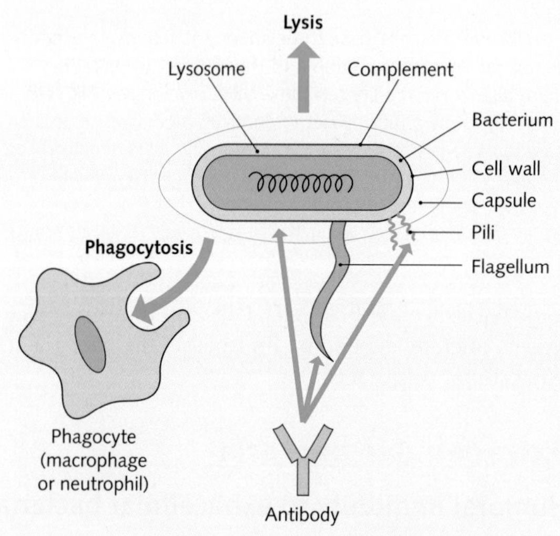

Fig. 11.5 The immune response to extracellular bacteria. The first line of host defence against bacteria is lysozyme. This 'natural antibiotic' attacks *N*-acetyl muramic acid–*N*-acetyl glucosamine links in the bacterial cell wall. This, together with complement, leads to bacterial lysis. Antibody is produced against flagella (immobilizing) and pili (prevents attachment). Capsular polysaccharides can induce T-cell-independent antibody. Antibodies aid complement activation and phagocytosis of bacteria.

Intracellular bacteria

Humoral immunity to intracellular bacteria

The humoral mechanisms that are employed against extracellular bacteria will be used to try to prevent bacteria causing intracellular infection. However, they will not be effective once the infection is intracellular.

Cell-mediated immunity to intracellular bacteria

Cell-mediated immunity is very important in the defence against intracellular bacterial infections, such as those caused by *M. tuberculosis*:

- Macrophages attempt to phagocytose the bacteria. If the organisms persist, chronic inflammation will ensue. This can lead to delayed (type IV) hypersensitivity (see p. 119)
- Cells infected with bacteria can activate NK cells, which cause cytotoxicity and can activate macrophages
- $CD4^+$ T cells release cytokines that activate macrophages (Th1 help)
- $CD8^+$ T cells recognize antigens presented in conjunction with class I MHC molecules on the surface of infected cells and lyse these cells.

Examples of infection and bacterial strategies to avoid immunity

Bacterial strategies to avoid the immune response must allow one of the following:

- Prevent phagocytosis. This is achieved in a number of ways. Some bacteria have capsules that inhibit phagocytosis, e.g. *Streptococcus pneumoniae, Haemophilus* spp. Others kill phagocytes with toxins or neutralize IgG, preventing opsonization, e.g. *Staphylococcus* spp.
- Allow survival within phagocytes, e.g. *M. tuberculosis, Mycobacterium leprae, Toxoplasma* spp.
- Prevent complement activation e.g. *Staphylococcus* spp., *Streptococcus* spp., *Haemophilus* spp., *Pseudomonas* spp.
- Avoid recognition by the immune system. This can be done through polymorphism, e.g. *Streptococcus pneumoniae, Salmonella typhi*.

Like viruses, bacteria can be highly polymorphic. Bacteria of the same species can appear to be entirely different to the immune system.

Immune response to protozoal infection

Protozoa are microscopic, single-celled organisms. Fewer than 20 types of protozoa infect humans, although malaria, trypanosomes and *Leishmania* cause significant morbidity and mortality. Protozoa cause intracellular infection, have marked antigenic variation and are often immunosuppressive. They have complex lifecycles, with several different stages, and, therefore, present the immune system with a variety of challenges. Protozoal infection is often chronic, as the immune system is not very efficient at dealing with these organisms. Most of the pathology of protozoal disease is caused by the immune response.

Humoral immunity against protozoa

Complement and antibody are important during the extracellular stage of infection. This opsonizes the protozoa and can cause lysis or prevent infection.

Cell-mediated immunity against protozoa

- *Phagocytosis* by macrophages, monocytes and neutrophils is an important part of the immune response against protozoa
- *CD4$^+$ T cells* are activated in response to protozoal infection. T helper 1 cytokines, e.g. IL-2, IFN-γ, TNF-β, are considered protective
- *Cytotoxic CD8$^+$ T cells* are important in destroying protozoa that replicate within cells, e.g. the sporozoite stage of *Plasmodium falciparum* (which causes malaria)
- *NK cells and mast cells* are often activated in protozoal infection.

Examples of protozoal infection and evasion of the immune response

Protozoa have good mechanisms to prevent the initiation of an immune response. Strategies include:

- Escape into the cytoplasm following phagocytosis, e.g. *Trypanosoma cruzi*
- Prevention of complement actions, e.g. *Leishmania* spp.
- Gene switching to create antigen variation, e.g. trypanosomes
- Immunosuppression, e.g. trypanosomes.

Immune response to worms

Multicellular parasites and worms pose a different problem to the immune system, as they are too large to be phagocytosed by macrophages and neutrophils. These worms tend to live on mucosal surfaces, and the immune system tries to dispose of these parasites by facilitating their expulsion. The immune system does this by secreting toxic chemicals onto mucosal surfaces, stimulating an increase in mucus secretion and smooth muscle contraction, which together result in expulsion of the worm.

Mast cells are stationed in tissues and have a similar sentinel purpose, with respect to worm infection, as that performed by macrophages for other types of infection. Mast cells contain preformed granules and, when they recognize parasitic infection through cross-linkage of IgE or possibly Toll-like receptors, they degranulate, releasing their preformed granules and other rapidly synthesized chemicals onto the parasite. They also release proinflammatory cytokines that recruit eosinophils and basophils.

Mast cell preformed granules contain:

- Histamine: causes smooth muscle in the walls of the gut to contract (expel the worm) and smooth muscle of blood vessels to relax
- Proteolytic enzymes: activate the complement system including anaphylatoxins.

The rapidly synthesized chemicals include prostaglandins and leukotrienes, both of which cause vasodilatation and contraction of smooth muscle in gut and bronchial walls.

Eosinophils secrete chemicals similar to those secreted by mast cells, excluding histamine. In addition they secrete:

- Peroxidase that generates hypochlorous acid
- A cationic protein which damages the worm's outer layers and paralyses its nervous system
- A basic protein that also attacks the outer layers of the worm.

Mast cells can be activated by IgE and, although this probably evolved to deal with worm infections, it mediates allergy (type I hypersensitivity).

Immune dysfunction

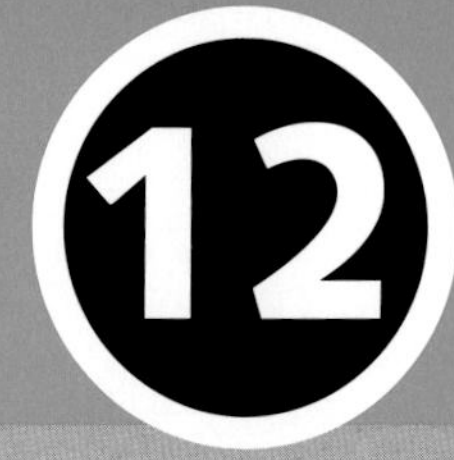

Objectives

You should be able to:

- Describe which processes lead to each form of hypersensitivity
- Outline the process of autoimmunity and how this leads to disease
- Explain the causes and features of immune deficiency
- Describe the immunological investigations of hypersensitivity, autoimmunity and immune deficiency.

HYPERSENSITIVITY

Concepts of hypersensitivity

Hypersensitivity is where there is an excessive and, therefore, inappropriate inflammatory response to any antigen. This inflammatory response results in tissue damage.

Hypersensitivity can occur in response to:

- An infection that cannot be cleared, e.g. tuberculosis
- A normally harmless exogenous substance, e.g. pollen
- An autoantigen, e.g. DNA in systemic lupus erythematosus (SLE).

Hypersensitivity reactions have been classified, by Gell and Coombs, into four types: I, II, III and IV. Types I, II and III are antibody-mediated; type IV is cell-mediated. In this system, the different types of hypersensitivity are classified by their time of onset after exposure to antigen.

Type I hypersensitivity (immediate hypersensitivity, allergy)

Type I hypersensitivity is mediated by IgE, with resultant and immediate degranulation of mast cells and basophils.

Overproduction of IgE in response to an innocuous environmental antigen occurs in allergy (see p. 120). Individuals with a greater inherited tendency towards type I hypersensitivity reactions are said to be atopic.

Type I hypersensitivity reactions require an initial antigen exposure in order to sensitize the immune system. When atopic individuals are exposed to an allergen they produce lots of IgE specific for that antigen. Mast cells have membrane receptors specific for the Fc portion of IgE, so that mast cells become coated in IgE. The immune system in now said to be sensitized to the allergen. Subsequent exposure to the same antigen, cross-linking mast cell surface IgE, results in release of preformed mediators of inflammation (degranulation). Short-lived basophils with IgE receptors are recruited and also degranulate in response to the antigen.

Mast cells and basophils release their contents within minutes of exposure to an allergen; this is the early phase response. The late phase response, mediated by eosinophils, responds to the same stimulus. This delay occurs as eosinophils have to be mobilized from the bone marrow. Clinically this can manifest itself as a further deterioration in symptoms several hours after initial exposure.

The immune mechanisms of type I reactions are illustrated in Fig. 12.1. Examples of type I reactions include:

- Allergic rhinitis (hay fever): pollens
- Allergic asthma: house-dust mite
- Systemic anaphylaxis: penicillin, peanuts or insect venom.

HINTS AND TIPS

Atopy is a genetic predisposition to produce IgE in response to many common, naturally occurring allergens. It has a prevalence of 10–30%. Atopic patients can suffer from multiple allergies. Atopy tends to run in families, however the genetic basis of atopy is not known.

When diagnosing type I hypersensitivity, the most important source of information is the history and the timing of events as the effects of allergy occur rapidly—within minutes. Allergy can result in a wide spectrum of symptoms, the most severe being anaphylaxis. This occurs as a consequence of increased vascular permeability and dilatation, causing large amounts of

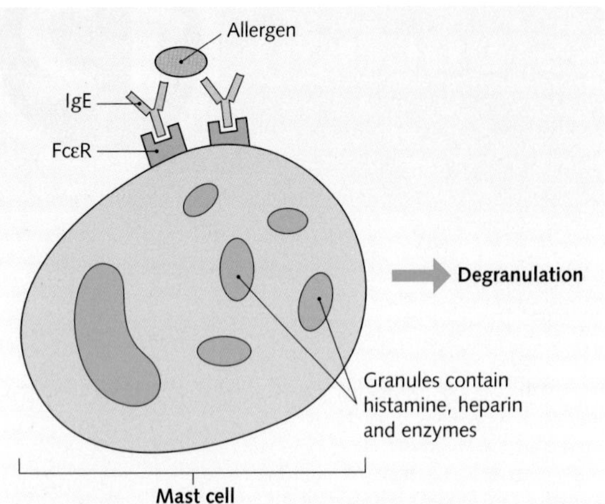

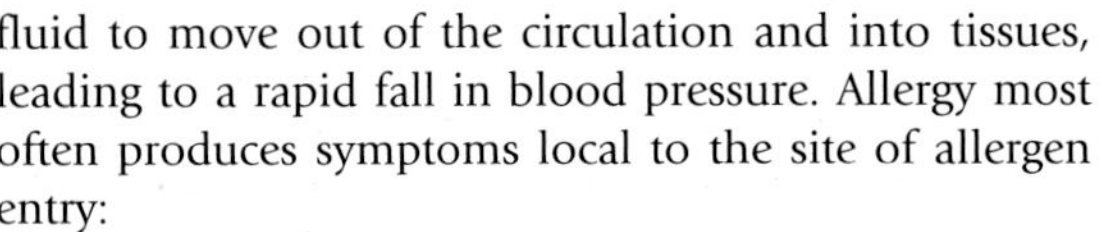

Fig. 12.1 The immune mechanisms of type I hypersensitivity reactions. Cross-linkage of IgE bound to cell surface receptors on mast cells and basophils results in degranulation.

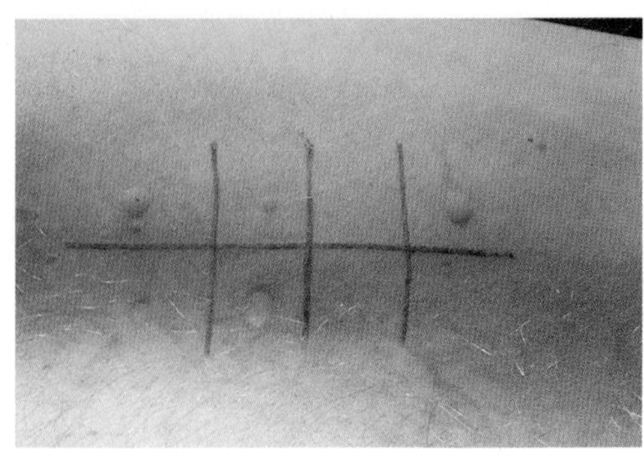

Fig 12.2 Skin prick testing. The presence of an itchy wheal, in a short amount of time, indicates a positive result. Reading clockwise from the top right: Positive control, negative contol, hazelnut, peanut, soya, peas, almond, cashew nut. This patient is allergic to peanut, soya, peas, almonds but not to hazelnut or cashew nut.

fluid to move out of the circulation and into tissues, leading to a rapid fall in blood pressure. Allergy most often produces symptoms local to the site of allergen entry:

- Skin: results in an urticarial rash or eczema
- Nasal mucosa: results in rhinitis, e.g. hay fever
- Lungs: can result in asthma.

For an allergic reaction to occur, IgE against that specific allergen needs to be present. This can be tested for using skin prick testing (this is not advisable for severe allergy) where a small amount of the suspected allergen is inoculated into the skin together with a positive and a negative control. A positive reaction will result in an itchy red lesion with a weal at the centre; the reaction is strongest after 15–20 minutes, indicating that the patient produces IgE to the tested allergen. Serum IgE can also be directly measured using a blood test.

Skin prick testing

A skin prick test is a useful way of assessing whether a person has IgE to different allergens (see Fig. 12.2). The response should always be compared to a histamine control.

Type II hypersensitivity

Type II (or antibody-mediated) hypersensitivity occurs when antibody specific for cell surface antigens is produced. Cell destruction can then result via:

- Complement activation
- Antibody-dependent cell-mediated cytotoxicity (ADCC)
- Phagocytosis.

The immune mechanisms of type II hypersensitivity reactions are summarized in Fig. 12.3.

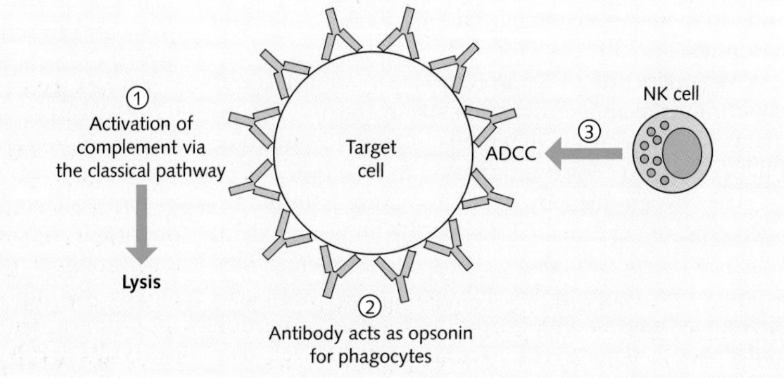

Fig. 12.3 The immune mechanisms of type II hypersensitivity reactions. Antibody bound to cells (either antibody to foreign cells or autoantibody) results in cell death via (1) complement, (2) phagocytes or (3) natural killer (NK) cells. ADCC, antibody-dependent cell-mediated cytotoxicity.

Examples of type II reactions in which complement is activated and cells destroyed are:

- Incompatible blood transfusions
- Haemolytic disease of the newborn
- Autoimmune haemolytic anaemias.

Some foreign antigens are too small to stimulate an immune response themselves, but need to bind to a host protein first. These antigens are called haptens. An example of a hapten involved in type II hypersensitivity is penicillin-induced haemolysis. Penicillin is too small to induce antibodies alone, but binds to the surface of red cells. It now acts as a hapten, inducing IgG production. The IgG then binds to the red cells, which leads to their destruction in the spleen.

Several diseases are caused by antibody directed against cell surface receptors, which can stimulate or block the receptor. In Graves' disease, stimulating antibodies are directed against the receptor for thyroid stimulating hormone. In myasthenia gravis, antibodies are directed against the acetylcholine receptor. They can destroy the receptor or cause lysis due to complement activation.

Type III hypersensitivity (immune complex)

Antibodies react to soluble (free) antigen by forming lattices of antibody and antigen, called an immune complex. This is a physiological response and is useful, for example, in the removal of bacterial exotoxin. The immune complexes are broken up by complement and transported to the spleen by red blood cells (RBCs) where they are phagocytosed. If there is a rapid influx in antigen that overwhelms these coping strategies, then a type III hypersensitivity reaction occurs (Fig. 12.4).

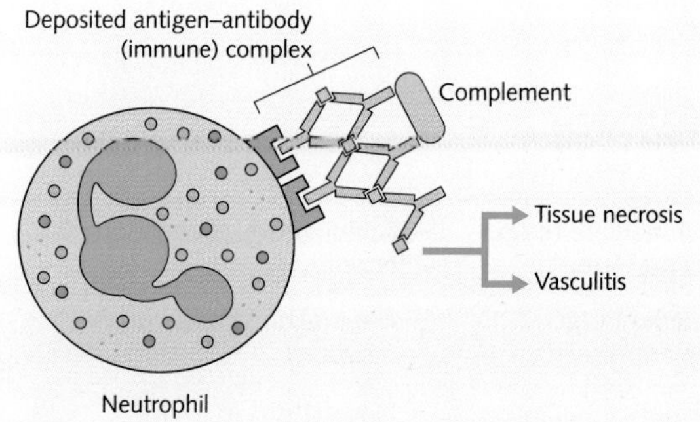

Fig. 12.4 The immune mechanisms of type III hypersensitivity reactions. Immune complexes that are normally removed by phagocytes are deposited in blood vessels or the tissues resulting in severe damage via complement and neutrophils.

HINTS AND TIPS

Type II hypersensitivity is based on antibodies (IgG) binding to cell-surface antigens, resulting in cell destruction. However, type III hypersensitivity occurs when antibodies bind free antigen. They form immune complexes that can cause tissue damage if present in excessive amounts.

Type III hypersensitivity can occur locally or systemically. Examples of local type III hypersensitivity include:

- Arthus reaction: intradermal or subcutaneous injection of antigen into a recipient with high levels of appropriate circulating antibody produces localized immune complexes that activate complement and generate acute inflammation
- Farmer's lung: inhalation of mould spores
- Pigeon fancier's disease: repeated inhalation of dried pigeon faeces.

Systemic type III hypersensitivity reactions occur when there is a large amount of antibody present throughout the body; this can occur when antigens such as antibiotics are injected into the circulation, or if the antigen is a self-antigen (an autoimmune reaction) such as occurs in SLE. Post-streptococcal glomerulonephritis is another important, systemic type III hypersensivity reaction. Antigen produced by *β-haemolytic streptococcus*, often after causing a sore throat, forms antigen-antibody complexes. These complexes produce inflammation in the glomeruli (glomerulonephritis).

Systemic lupus erythematosus (SLE)

In immune complex disease in general, and SLE in particular, immune complexes precipitate out in the glomeruli, skin and joints, leading to characteristic clinical signs.

Type IV hypersensitivity (delayed)

Upon first contact with antigen, a subset of $CD4^+$ T helper (Th) cells is activated and clonally expanded (this takes 1–2 weeks). Upon subsequent encounter with the same antigen, sensitized Th cells secrete cytokines. These attract and activate macrophages, which account for more than 95% of the cells involved. Activated macrophages have increased phagocytic ability and can destroy pathogens more effectively. The type IV reaction peaks at 48–72 hours after contact with the antigen (time taken for the recruitment and activation of the macrophages) and is therefore known as delayed-type

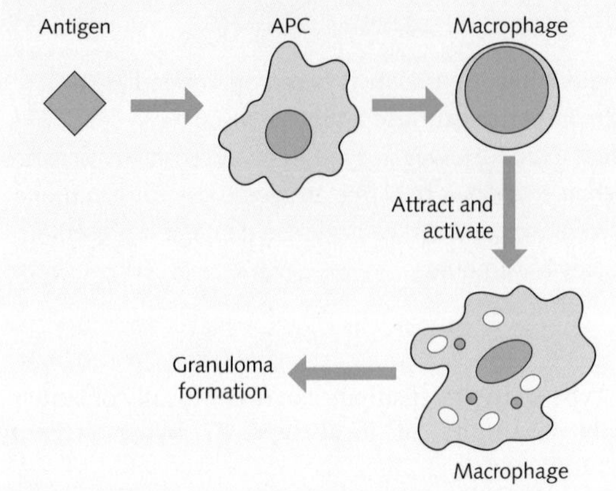

Fig. 12.5 The immune mechanisms of type IV hypersensitivity reactions. These reactions take several days to be initiated because antigen is first presented to T cells, which can then activate macrophages. APC, antigen-presenting cell.

hypersensitivity. An overview of the immune mechanisms involved is given in Fig. 12.5.

Type IV reactions are important for the clearance of intracellular pathogens. However, if antigen persists, the response can be detrimental to the individual, as the lytic products of the activated macrophages can damage healthy tissues. Examples of antigens that induce a type IV response are:

- Contact dermatitis to antigens such as nickel
- Intracellular pathogens such as *M. tuberculosis*.

As with type I reactions skin testing is used to detect type IV reactions. Instead of a skin prick, however, patch testing is used to diagnose antigens causing delayed hypersensitivity in contact dermatitis. A selection of sensitizing antigens are normally tested at the same time. They are usually placed in a grid pattern on the upper back and then dressed. Patients are then seen, sometimes more than once, over the next 48–72 hours to assess the response. The response varies from no response to an extreme reaction.

The tuberculin skin test can be used to determine whether a person has been exposed to *M. tuberculosis*. An intradermal injection of purified protein derivative (PPD) is given to the individual. Previous exposure to *M. tuberculosis* or bacille Calmette–Guérin (BCG) vaccination results in a positive response. This is apparent as a firm, red (due to the intense infiltration of macrophages) lesion at the injection site 48–72 hours after the injection. The skin lesions in both contact dermatitis and tuberculin testing are composed of macrophages and T cells.

A summary of the four types of hypersensitivity is shown in Fig. 12.6.

ALLERGY

Allergy is due to immediate hypersensitivity reactions to exogenous antigens (known as allergens), mediated by IgE. Allergic symptoms usually result from degranulation of mast cells, mediated by the cross-linking of IgE by allergen. Allergic conditions are therefore type I hypersensitivity reactions. The symptoms of different allergies affect different tissues and can be local or generalized.

Asthma

Asthma is a chronic inflammatory disorder of the airways, characterized by reversible airflow obstruction. The airways become hyper-responsive and exaggerated bronchoconstriction follows a wide variety of non-immunological stimuli, e.g. exercise or cold air. The symptoms of asthma are cough, wheeze, chest tightness and shortness of breath. Asthma is a common disease and is diagnosed in 5–10% of children. The incidence has risen over the last few decades, particularly in more economically developed countries.

Fig. 12.6 Summary of the different types of hypersensitivity

Type of hypersensitivity	Immune mediators	Time of onset	Examples
Type I	IgE, mast cells, eosinophils	Immediate (if IgE is preformed)	Anaphylaxis, asthma, atopic eczema
Type II	Antibody (normally IgG), complement, phagocytes	Rapid (if IgG is preformed)	Haemolytic disease of the newborn, ABO incompatibility
Type III	IgG, complement and neutrophils	Hours	SLE, arthrus reaction
Type IV	Th cells, macrophages	48–72 hours	Contact dermatitis, tuberculin skin test

SLE, systemic lupus erythematosus; Th cells, T helper cells.

Pollens, house-dust mite faeces and animal fur are the most common allergens. These cause inflammation of the bronchial wall involving:

- Infiltration by eosinophils, mast cells, lymphocytes and neutrophils
- Oedema of the submucosa
- Smooth muscle hypertrophy and hyperplasia
- Thickening of the basement membrane
- Mucous plugging
- Epithelial desquamation.

Asthma is diagnosed by a reversal in airway obstruction (measured by peak expiratory flow rate, or 'peak flow') of $\geq$15%, either spontaneously or following the administration of an inhaled short-acting β_2-adrenoreceptor agonist (such as salbutamol). Advice including avoidance of triggers and how to manage an attack should be given. Short-acting β_2-adrenoreceptor agonists are used as the treatment for short-term improvement of symptoms, although inhaled steroids and other immunosuppressive/anti-inflammatory drugs are used prophylactically to prevent asthma attacks. This is as per the British Thoracic Society's step-wise approach.

Allergic rhinitis

Nasal congestion, watery nasal discharge and sneezing occur after exposure to allergen. The most common allergens are grass, flower, weed or tree pollens, which cause a seasonal rhinitis (hay fever), and house-dust mite faeces, which can cause a more perennial rhinitis. Allergic attacks usually last for a few hours and are often accompanied by itching and watering of the eyes. Skin prick tests can identify the allergen.

The most important treatment is topical (nasal) steroids; alternatives or adjuncts include antihistamines or mast cell stabilizers such as sodium cromoglicate. Avoidance of allergens is advised but is often difficult.

Atopic/allergic eczema

Eczema or dermatitis can be caused by an allergic response. Dermatitis means skin inflammation. There are several types of dermatitis, including allergic (atopic) eczema (type I hypersensitivity reaction) and contact dermatitis (a type IV hypersensitivity reaction). Contact dermatitis can be diagnosed by patch testing and treatment is primarily by avoidance of the antigen (e.g. nickel).

Atopic eczema is most commonly the result of exposure to pollen or house-dust mite faeces. Common allergens are shown in Fig. 12.7. About 10% of children are diagnosed with eczema. Eczema commonly affects the flexural creases and the fronts of the wrist and ankles. In infancy and adulthood the face and trunk are often involved. The skin lesions are itchy, red, sometimes vesicular and might be dry. Because of itching, the skin is often excoriated, which can lead to lichenification

Fig. 12.7 Summary of allergic reactions

Allergic condition	Common allergens	Features
Systemic anaphylaxis	Drugs Serum Venoms Peanuts	Oedema with increased vascular permeability Leads to tracheal occlusion, circulatory collapse and possibly death
Allergic rhinitis	Pollen (hay fever) Dust-mite faeces (perennial rhinitis)	Sneezing, oedema and irritation of nasal mucosa
Asthma	Pollen Dust-mite faeces	Bronchial constriction, increased mucus production, airway inflammation
Food	Shellfish Milk Eggs Fish Wheat	Itching urticaria and potentially anaphylaxis
Atopic eczema	Pollen Dust-mite faeces Some foods	Itchy inflammation of the skin

(thickening of the skin). Eczema is often complicated by superinfection with bacteria, particularly *Staphylococcus aureus*.

Recently, mutations in a gene encoding for Filaggrin (a protein that binds to keratin fibres in epithelial cells) has been associated with atopic eczema.

The diagnosis of atopic eczema is usually clinical. Total serum IgE, RAST for specific IgE and skin prick testing with common allergens are occasionally performed to confirm the diagnosis of atopic eczema. Treatment of eczema is mainly topical, except in more severe cases, when systemic steroids and immunosuppressants are used. Therapies include:

- Emollients: moisturizes dry skin and reduces itching
- Topical steroids: anti-inflammatory
- Topical antibiotics or antiseptics: in infected eczema
- Oral antihistamine: reduces itching
- Ciclosporin: resistant cases might require immunosuppression.

Anaphylaxis

Anaphylaxis is a medical emergency and can be fatal. However, it is rapidly reversible if treated properly. A systemic response to an allergen that is either intravenous or rapidly absorbed can cause laryngeal occlusion and shock. Many allergens can cause anaphylaxis, but more common environmental causes include bee stings and peanuts. Many cases of anaphylaxis take place in hospital where they can be triggered by antibiotics or latex. The signs of anaphylaxis are principally those of shock. Signs include:

- Hypotension with tachycardia
- Warm peripheral temperature
- Signs of airway obstruction
- Laryngeal and facial oedema and urticaria (often seen).

The management of anaphylaxis, as per the Resuscitation Council (UK) guidelines, should be known by all medical professionals. The initial management of anaphylaxis is resuscitation, i.e. attend to life-threatening airway, breathing and/or circulatory problems. Allergens should be removed if possible, e.g. stop drug infusion. Adrenaline (epinephrine) should be given as soon as possible, intramuscularly (IM). The dose for adults is 0.5 mL of 1:1000, and should be repeated after 5 minutes if there is no improvement. Adrenaline should be given intravenously only by a specialist and in environments where monitoring is possible, and at a lower dose. An intravenous (IV) fluid challenge of between 500 and 1000 mL should be given next, to correct hypotension. Chloramphenamine (an anti-histamine) and hydrocortisone are also given later in the management.

HINTS AND TIPS

Any patient that suffers from a proven or suspected anaphylactic reaction should be seen in an allergy clinic by a specialist. They should receive advice regarding future attacks, as well as training on how to administer intramuscular adrenaline. They should carry a preloaded adrenaline syringe for such occasions.

AUTOIMMUNITY

Prevention of autoimmunity

Autoimmunity is a state in which the body exhibits immunological reactivity to itself. 'Self-tolerance' is the generic term given to the mechanisms by which T and B cells are prevented from responding to self. Because T and B cells randomly recombine the genes for their receptors, there is a risk of producing receptors that will react with self-antigen. These cells must be eliminated to make the host tolerant to itself.

Central tolerance

Central tolerance is by negative selection—early clonal deletion. T cells (in the thymus) and B cells (in the bone marrow) are eliminated if they are self-reactive. Central tolerance is not complete. Only the most self-reactive lymphocytes are deleted, ensuring that a wide lymphocyte repertoire is maintained.

Peripheral tolerance

In the periphery, self-antigens do not generally elicit an immune response. Several mechanisms prevent self-reactive T cells from causing autoimmune disease, including:

- Lack of the co-stimulatory molecules required for T cell activation, e.g. CD40 or CD28 or low level MHC expression
- Sequestration of the antigen behind a physical barrier, e.g. the testis
- T cells entering immune privileged sites undergo apoptosis (via Fas, transforming growth factor (TGF)-β or IL-10). Immune privileged sites include the brain, testis and the anterior chamber of the eye
- There is also a specialist population of regulatory T cells (Tregs) which are able to suppress immune responses to self.

Causes of autoimmunity—breakdown of tolerance

If tolerance breaks down, autoimmunity can develop. Tolerance can break down in the thymus (usually for genetic reasons) or in the periphery (usually as a result of environmental factors such as infection). Autoimmunity is multifactorial; a defect in at least one of the regulatory mechanisms is required before disease develops.

Role of human leucocyte antigen (HLA)—genetic predisposition

Many autoimmune diseases have a familial component. The HLA haplotype is the main identified genetic factor. If an individual has inherited an HLA allele that does not bind self-antigen with high affinity, reactive T cells are not deleted in the thymus. Certain HLA alleles are linked to specific autoimmune processes, e.g. HLA-DR4 in rheumatoid arthritis, and HLA-DQ8 in coeliac disease. However, a certain HLA haplotype does not automatically result in the development of an autoimmune disease; 95% of patients with ankylosing spondylitis have HLA-B27, but only 5% of the population with HLA-B27 have ankylosing spondylitis.

Role of infection—polyclonal activation

Many infections are able to activate T and B cells in a non-specific fashion. This results in the proliferation of several T and B cell clones, which can produce autoreactive autoantibody or mediate autoimmunity.

Role of infection—inappropriate MHC expression

Infection stimulates antigen-presenting cells (APC), and the upregulation of MHC class II molecules. This can result in activation of autoreactive T cells.

Mechanisms of autoimmunity

Autoimmune diseases are hypersensitivity reactions in which an exaggerated response is triggered by self-antigen. Autoimmune diseases can therefore be classified in the same way as hypersensitivity (excluding type I hypersensitivity).

Antibody-mediated (type II hypersensitivity reactions)

Antibodies that are specific for self-antigen bind to tissues or cells. Autoimmunity can result from a variety of mechanisms, including:

- Opsonization: e.g. in autoimmune haemolytic anaemia, IgG binds to red blood cells, which are phagocytosed by macrophages in the spleen
- Complement activation: e.g. in severe autoimmune haemolytic anaemia, IgM antibodies bound to red blood cells activate complement, resulting in lysis within the circulation.

Neutralization and ADCC can also occur in response to self-antigen.

Immune-complex-mediated (type III hypersensitivity reactions)

Immune complexes are lattices of antigen and antibody. They are usually cleared rapidly from the circulation, but complexes that are not cleared trigger inflammation, particularly in blood vessels. An example of a type III autoimmune disease is SLE. A consequence of the presence of circulating immune complexes can be the development of glomerulonephritis. Immune complexes deposit in the capillaries of the glomerular tufts in the kidneys, resulting in renal failure. Immune complexes are also deposited at other sites, e.g. joints, skin and brain.

Cell-mediated (type IV hypersensitivity reactions)

These comprise autoimmune T cell responses, usually by T helper and T cytotoxic cells. Examples include rheumatoid arthritis and type I diabetes mellitus.

Clinically autoimmunity is divided into systemic (connective tissue diseases and vasculitis) and organ-specific conditions.

Systemic autoimmune diseases

Systemic lupus erythematosus (SLE)

Patients with SLE often have autoantibodies directed against DNA, histone proteins, red blood cells, platelets, leucocytes and clotting factors. However, some of these autoantibodies are also seen in other autoimmune conditions. The most specific for SLE is anti-double stranded DNA (anti-dsDNA). Diagnosis is by antinuclear antibody testing. It is most commonly diagnosed in women in the second or third decade of life.

The aetiology is unknown but the vast array of autoantibodies present suggests a breakdown of self-tolerance. Genetic factors predispose to the disease. There is an association with HLA-DR2 and HLA-DR3, and with deficiencies of complement proteins, especially C2 or C4 (reduced complement levels result in a decreased ability to clear immune complexes). Other relevant aetiological factors include drugs such as hydralazine, exposure to ultraviolet light and oestrogens.

Deposition of immune complexes leads to the various clinical features of SLE, including:

- Arthritis (deposition in joints)
- Rashes in sun-exposed areas
- Glomerulonephritis.

SLE is treated with immunosuppression, steroids, NSAIDs or other anti-inflammatory drugs.

Rheumatoid arthritis (RA)

HINTS AND TIPS

A typical feature of rheumatoid arthritis is joint pain and stiffness on waking that lasts at least 30 minutes.

RA is a chronic systemic disease that primarily involves the joints, resulting in inflammation of the synovium and destruction of the articular cartilage (Fig. 12.8). Initially, the disease affects the small joints of the hands and feet symmetrically, later spreading to the larger joints. RA affects approximately 1–2% of the

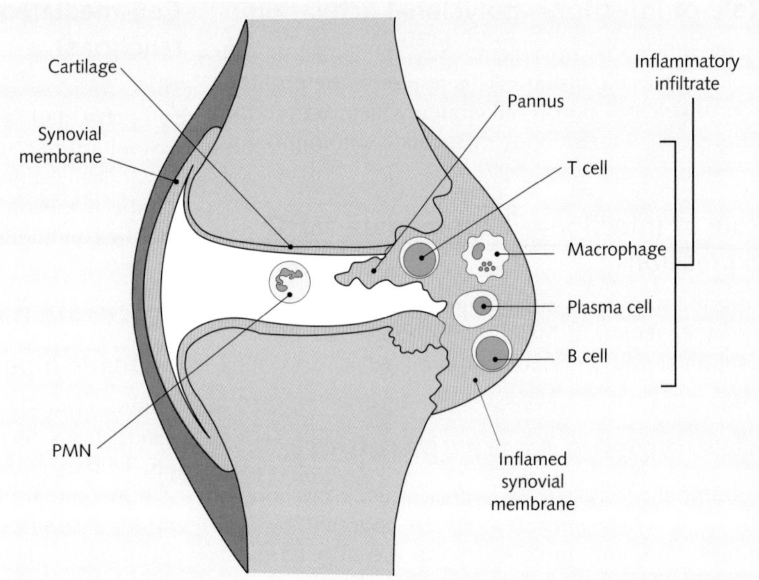

Fig. 12.8 Rheumatoid joint showing pannus formation and cartilage destruction. The synovial membrane is infiltrated by inflammatory cells and hypertrophies to form granulation tissue known as 'pannus'. This eventually erodes the articular cartilage and bone. T cells and macrophages in the inflamed synovium secrete tumour necrosis factor. PMN, polymorphonuclear neutrophil.

world's population and is most common between the ages of 30 and 55 years. The female:male ratio is 3:1.

Approximately 70% of RA patients carry either the HLA-DR4 or HLA-DR1 haplotype. The immunopathogenesis of RA is outlined in Fig. 12.9.

A key event in RA is secretion of TNF by T cells and macrophages, which causes joint inflammation and erosion of bone. Once RA is suspected clinically, prompt referral is essential to minimize morbidity associated with this chronic condition. Management is based on early use of steroids and non-steroidal anti-inflammatories (NSAIDs). Specific anti-rheumatic drugs that modulate the immune response, known as disease-modifying antirheumatic drugs (DMARDs), are also used. These DMARDs usually target TNF (e.g. infliximab and etanercept). The anti-B cell monoclonal antibody rituximab is also used.

Rheumatoid arthritis – investigations

The blood tests in RA reflect its inflammatory nature; CRP and ESR are raised, indicating an acute phase response. Rheumatoid nodules are present when the patient has made IgM anti-IgG autoantibodies (rheumatoid factor) and indicate a poorer prognosis than those who are rheumatoid factor negative. RF is positive in approximately 80% of RA patients.

Radiographic features include:

- Soft tissue swelling
- Juxta-articular osteoporosis
- Joint space narrowing
- Joint destruction and erosions (see Fig. 12.10)
- Subluxation.

A summary of other systemic connective tissue disorders and vasculitides is given in Figs 12.11 and 12.12.

HINTS AND TIPS

Other autoantibodies associated with specific diseases include:

- Anti-smooth muscle antibody—chronic autoimmune hepatitis
- Anti-mitochondrial antibody (AMA)—primary biliary cirrhosis.

Wegener's granulomatosis

Wegener's granulomatosis is a systemic vasculitis (results from blood vessel inflammation) that affects the nose, lungs and kidneys. The pathogenesis of Wegener's is linked to antibodies directed against proteinase-3, an enzyme present in the cytoplasm of neutrophils (c-ANCA). It causes neutrophils to become trapped in vessel walls where they release proinflammatory cytokines and cause damage. The most severe complication

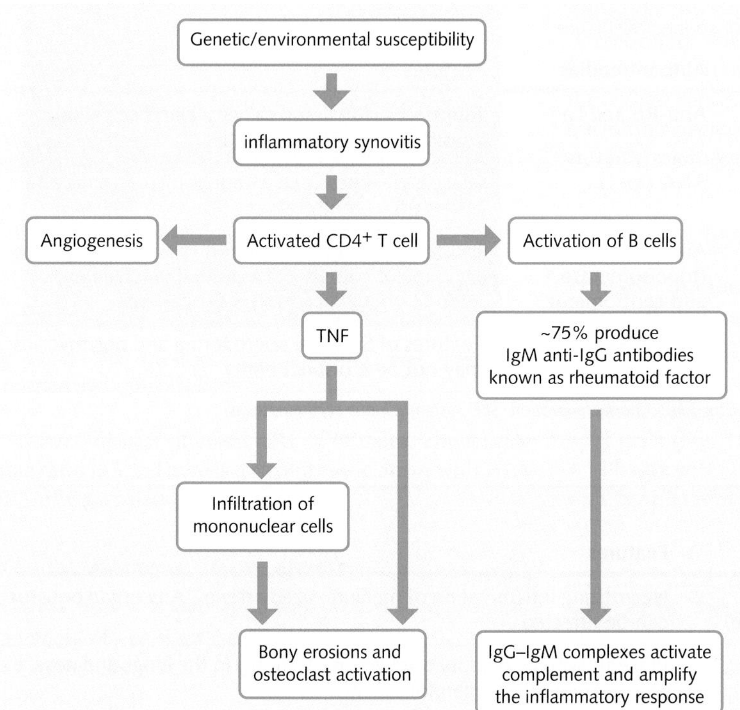

Fig. 12.9 Pathogenesis of rheumatoid arthritis (RA). Autoreactive $CD4^+$ T cells mediate the pathological changes. Synovial T cells produce a number of cytokines including tumour necrosis factor (TNF). These stimulate the acute phase response, synovial inflammation and bone erosion. Activation of B cells can result in the production of rheumatoid factor and immune complex formation.

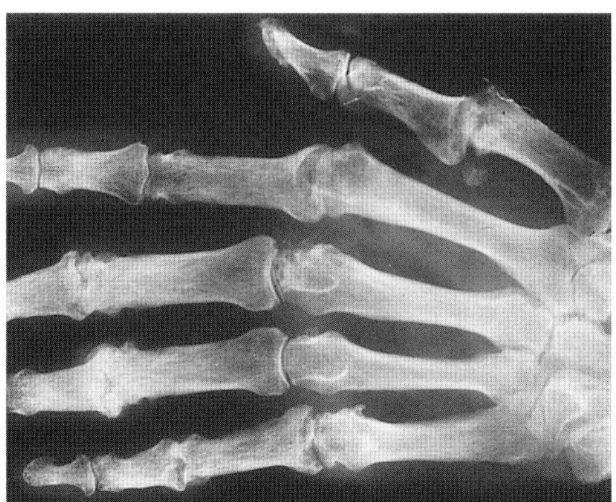

Fig. 12.10 A hand X-ray showing joint destruction and erosions due to rhuematoid arthritis.

is kidney failure; however, the use of immunosuppressives has drastically improved the prognosis.

Organ- or cell-type-specific autoimmune diseases

A summary of organ- or cell-type-specific diseases is given in Fig. 12.13.

Hashimoto's thyroiditis

Hashimoto's thyroiditis is the most common cause of goitrous hypothyroidism (although there is also an atrophic form). Antigen-specific cytotoxic T cells attack the thyroid gland, leading to progressive destruction of the epithelium. Marked lymphocytic infiltration (mainly by B cells and $CD4^+$ T cells) of the thyroid gland is accompanied by migration of large numbers of macrophages and plasma cells, resulting in the formation of lymphoid follicles and germinal centres within the thyroid. Due to unregulated T-helper cell interaction with B cells, autoantibodies are produced against thyroid antigens such as thyroid peroxidase.

Middle-aged females are most commonly affected (female:male ratio as high as 20:1). The disease is associated with the HLA-DR5 haplotype.

Graves' disease

Graves' disease is the commonest cause of hyperthyroidism. This arises as a result of IgG autoantibody production against the thyroid stimulating hormone receptor that actively stimulates the receptor, resulting in increased thyroxine production.

Fig. 12.16 Primary lymphocyte deficiencies

Disorder	Features
DiGeorge syndrome (thymic hypoplasia)	Intrauterine damage to the third and fourth pharyngeal pouches results in failure of development of the thyroid and parathyroid glands. This results in a decrease in the number and function of T cells Clinical features include abnormal facies, cardiac defects, hypoparathyroidism and recurrent infections
Severe combined immunodeficiency disease (SCID)	Lymphocyte deficiency and failure of thymic development due to inherited abnormalities: • X-linked SCID is due to defects in the γ-chain of the IL-2 receptor. The γ-chain forms part of several cytokine receptors including IL-7, which is needed for T cell maturation • Autosomal recessive SCID is caused by defects in adenosine deaminase (ADA) or purine nucleoside phosphorylase in more than 50% of cases. Both are involved in purine degradation and deficiency results in accumulation of toxic metabolites and inhibition of DNA synthesis. Recombinase defects also lead to SCID In both types of SCID, treatment should be by bone marrow transplant, usually before the age of 2 years. Trials using gene therapy to treat X-linked SCID were stopped due to an increased risk of leukaemia
Wiskott–Aldrich syndrome	X-linked recessive condition characterized by normal serum IgG, low IgM and high IgA and IgE. Defective T cell function is seen, which worsens as the patient ages. Patients tend to get recurrent infections, eczema and thrombocytopenia

Primary lymphocyte deficiencies include infections with opportunistic pathogens such as Pneumocystis carinii. T cell deficiency can cause an antibody deficiency due to lack of T-helper-cell activation of B cells.

Fig. 12.17 Primary phagocyte deficiencies

Disorder	Features
Neutropenia	See p. 43
Leucocyte adhesion deficiency	Lack of β_2-integrin molecules results in impaired adhesion and extravasation of phagocytes
Chronic granulomatous disease	Most commonly X-linked (can be autosomal recessive) inheritance. Lack of NADPH oxidase impairs killing of ingested pathogens, which therefore persist. Can be tested by impaired reduction of nitroblue tetrazolium by stimulated neutrophils

NADPH, nicotinamide adenine dinucleotide phosphate.

Fig. 12.18 Primary complement deficiencies

Disorder	Features
Deficiency of classical pathway components	Tend to develop immune complex disease
C3 deficiency	Prone to recurrent pyogenic infections
Deficiency of C5, C6, C 7, C8, factor D, properdin	Increased susceptibility to *Neisseria* infections
C1 inhibitor deficiency	Causes hereditary angioedema

Deficiencies of almost all complement components have been described.

HINTS AND TIPS

Any patient presenting with a **S**erious, **P**ersistent, **U**nusual or **R**ecurrent infection should **SPUR** a clinician to think about immunodeficiency.

It is important to recognize primary immunodeficiencies. Patients with an antibody deficiency will develop irreversible lung infections (bronchiectasis) unless given immunoglobulin. Children with T cell defects can be killed by opportunistic infections or from live vaccines such as BCG.

Neonates do not possess a fully developed immune system at birth. In the neonatal period, infants are normally protected by maternal IgG that crossed the placenta in utero, but this is metabolized during the first months of life. Infants normally begin production of their own IgG by 3 months (Fig. 12.19). In some individuals, IgG production might not start for up to 9–12 months, possibly due to lack of help from T cells.

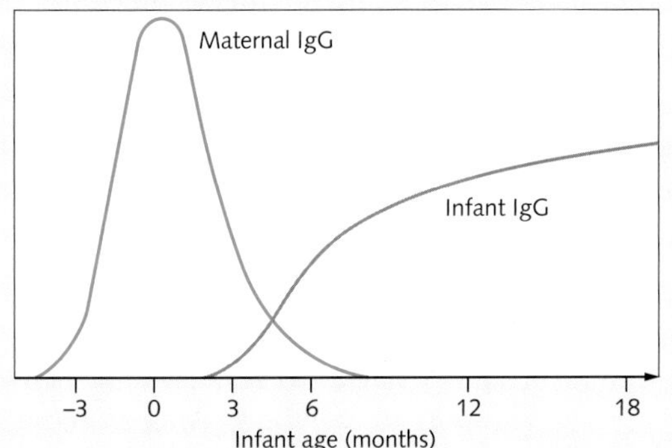

Fig. 12.19 Plasma levels of maternal and neonatal immunoglobulin in the normal-term infant. In the first 6 months of life there is a trough in immunoglobulin levels that makes infants prone to infection. IgA in breast milk can compensate. Babies born prematurely are deprived of maternal IgG and suffer exaggerated neonatal antibody deficiency.

HINTS AND TIPS

Mutations in the the gene for one of the pattern recognition molecules, nucleotide-binding oligomerization domain containing 2 (NOD2) gene are important in some cases of inflammatory bowel disease (IBD), and especially Crohn's disease. For many years, Crohn's disease was thought to be autoimmune. Now it appears that some cases are caused by defects in the innate immune system.

Secondary immune deficiencies

Malnutrition and disease

Rarely, lack of dietary protein and certain elements (e.g. zinc) predisposes to secondary immunodeficiency. Infections such as malaria and measles also result in immunodeficiency.

Malignancy

Secondary immunodeficiency is particularly common with tumours that arise from the immune system, such as myeloma, lymphoma and leukaemia (see Chapter 5). Many other tumours are immunosuppressive. This is likely to provide the tumour cells with a selective advantage, because they evade destruction by cytotoxic cells.

Steroids, other drugs and radiation

Iatrogenic causes of immunosuppression are common. Immunosuppressive drugs can be given to suppress inflammatory or autoimmune disease, or to prevent rejection of transplanted material (see p. 137). Radiation and cytotoxic drugs can be used to treat malignancies and frequently cause immunosuppression.

Acquired immunodeficiency syndrome (AIDS)

AIDS is caused by infection with HIV. HIV is a retrovirus, containing a small amount of RNA that codes three important viral genes: the envelope, reverse transcriptase and protease (Fig. 12.20).

The envelope is composed of gp120 which binds to CD4 receptors and chemokine receptor 5 (CCR5). A conformational change causes gp41 to be expressed, which penetrates the host cell. This process allows HIV to infect:

- CD4 T cells
- Monocytes and macrophages
- Dendritic cells.

Reverse transcriptase is an enzyme that catalyses the production of HIV DNA from viral RNA, using host cellular machinery.

Protease is an enzyme that cleaves proteins into their component peptides, and is important for viral assembly and activity.

Transmission of HIV

Sexual transmission is the most important route for spread; HIV infects mucosal macrophages and dendritic cells via CD4 and CC5. These professional APCs then aid in the evolution of the HIV infection by transporting

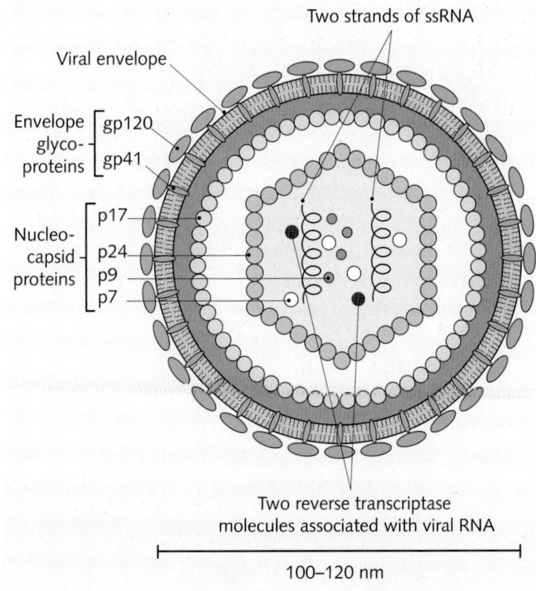

Fig. 12.20 Structure of HIV-1. The envelope glycoproteins gp120 and gp41 are hypervariable. gp120 binds CD4, while gp41 enables entry of the virus into the cell. The viral envelope is a lipid bilayer containing both viral glycoprotein antigens and host proteins.

it to the lymph nodes where HIV can gain easy access to CD4 T helper cells.

Transmission can also occur through infected blood: blood transfusions, intravenous drug abusers and needlestick injury (0.3% risk from a single exposure). These routes do not require HIV to gain access through mucous membranes and hence CC5 receptors. Vertical transmission is especially important in developing countries, occurring transplacentally during labour (approximately 25% of cases) or through breast milk.

Immune response to HIV

Most individuals exposed to HIV sexually become chronically infected. Infected individuals produce antibody, but this is largely ineffective against intracellular virus. T cells inhibit HIV (by interferon secretion) or kill infected cells.

The primary infection is often asymptomatic but may be marked by a flu-like illness (fever, macular rash, mouth ulcers, splenomegaly and diarrhoea) in 15% of individuals.

HIV seroconversion illness

Individuals infected with HIV develop symptoms as their body starts to produce antibody to HIV. This is called HIV seroconversion illness. The patient experiences fever, rash, malaise, sore throat, diarrhoea and arthralgia; lymphadenopathy may also be present. Not all patients experience seroconversion illness, and it is often diagnosed retrospectively.

How does HIV progress to AIDS?

1. Mutations: reverse transcriptase makes an error for roughly 1 in every 10,000 bases. Some of these mutations provide a selective advantage to the HIV, e.g. cells of the immune system may no longer recognize them, and another immune response has to start afresh.
2. Even if the immune system manages to clear the entire free virus, HIV can hide in host DNA and remain dormant for many years—the latent phase. Reactivation of the host cell then results in production of HIV RNA, and thus the infection continues.
3. HIV infects and destroys the cells that are responsible for the immune response. As the CD4 count declines, the cytotoxic T lymphocytes become less effective as they are receiving less support from T helper cells.

HINTS AND TIPS

Each infected individual contains many hundreds of slightly different strains following infection with a single virus.

Diagnosis and monitoring of an HIV infection

Screening for HIV infection is performed using enzyme-linked immunosorbent assays (ELISAs) to detect anti-HIV antibodies. If the ELISA is positive, confirmatory tests must be carried out, e.g. a Western blot, which detects antibodies against specific HIV proteins. As seroconversion (production of antibodies) might not take place until 3 months after infection, there is a window period when ELISA will be negative. This is a potential problem in blood transfusion.

In infants, anti-HIV IgG can be maternally derived and persist for up to 18 months, making diagnosis of HIV by ELISA unreliable. Detection of HIV by polymerase chain reaction (PCR) is used to confirm HIV infection in neonates.

HINTS AND TIPS

False positives may occur with the HIV enzyme-linked immunosorbent assay (ELISA) in those with recent influenza vaccination, hepatic disease or a recent viral infection.

Determinations of CD4 T cell counts and measurement of the viral load (serum HIV RNA) are useful in assessing response to treatment and the prognosis.

CD4 counts provide a guide of the current immunological status of the patient (Fig. 12.21), whereas HIV RNA levels predict what will happen to the patient over the next few months and years.

During the latent phase of the infection T cells are constantly battling with the HIV, and gradually the CD4 count falls. With the falling CD4 count, individuals become susceptible to more and more organisms. Initially these include virulent organisms such as *Candida albicans* and *Mycobacterium tuberculosis*. However, as the CD4 count continues to fall the individual is more susceptible to opportunistic infections (Figure 12.22). When the CD4 count drops to < 200 cells/μL or the individual begins to suffer from an infection indicative of AIDS (an 'AIDS-defining condition'), they are said to be suffering from AIDS (as opposed to just being HIV +ve).

HINTS AND TIPS

Individuals with HIV should have their CD4 and viral load levels checked every 3–6 months.

Treatment of HIV

The treatment of HIV is now very successful. Although the infection cannot be cured, survival and quality of life have been profoundly increased. The drugs used

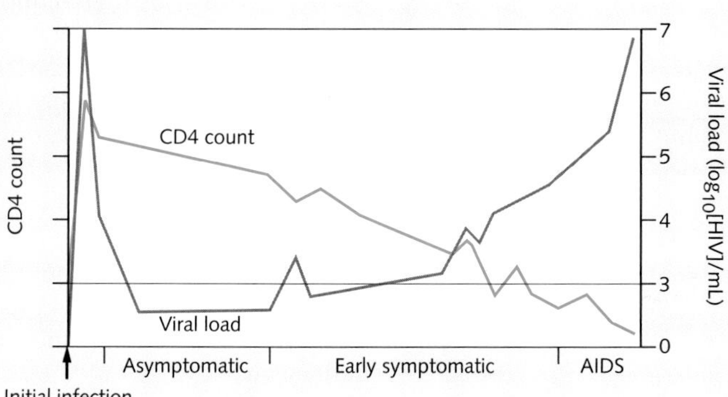

Fig. 12.21 Variation in CD4 count and viral load during the course of HIV infection.

Fig. 12.22 Clinical infections at different CD4 counts	
CD4 count	**Infection**
< 400	Tuberculosis
< 300	Kaposi's sarcoma. Oesophageal candidiasis
< 200	*Pneumocystis carinii* pneumonia (PCP) Toxoplasmosis
< 100	*Mycobacterium avium intracellulare* Cytomegalovirus retinitis

to combat the virus are termed antiretrovirals (ARVs) and include classes of drug that work on the three main elements of the virus (Fig. 12.23):

- Fusion inhibitors prevent attachment to the envelope
- Reverse transcriptase inhibitors (RTIs) inhibit the production of DNA. There are both nucleotide analogue RTIs (NARTIs) and non-nucleotide RTI (NNRTIs)
- Protease inhibitors prevent the production of viral peptides.

When treating HIV it is important to remember its ability to mutate and that antiretrovirals could provide

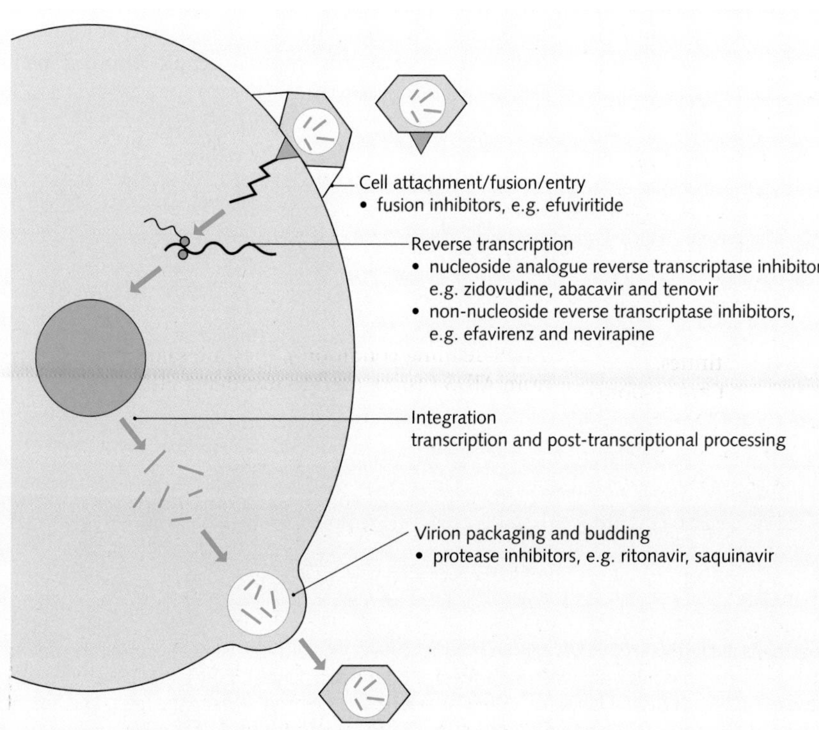

Fig. 12.23 Antiretroviral agents in current use and their site of action in the lifecycle of HIV.

a selective advantage for a more resistant strain to develop. For this reason a combination of a least two classes of drug are used and they are not started until there is evidence of CD4 T cell decline. This combination of more than one drug is known as highly active antiretroviral therapy (HAART).

Antibiotic prophylaxis against infections such as *Pneumocystis carinii* and *Toxoplasma gondii* is effective and usually given when the CD4 count is $< 200/\mu L$. It has been shown that antibiotic prophylaxis can be safely stopped following immune restoration using treatment with antiretroviral therapy.

Vertical transmission can be vastly reduced by:

- Delivering by Caesarean section
- Early antiretroviral use
- No breast feeding.

INVESTIGATION OF IMMUNE FUNCTION

Immunoassays

This is a technique that uses antibody to identify antigen or biological molecules.

Enzyme-linked immunosorbent assay (ELISA)

ELISA is a sensitive test that allows quantitative analysis of the amount of a specific antigen or antigen/antibody complex in a sample.

In an ELISA an enzyme is attached to the antigen under study, and catalyses the conversion of a colourless substrate to a coloured product. The amount of coloured end-product is proportional to the amount of antigen and can be measured using a spectrometer.

ELISAs are commonly used to measure specific antibody in a patient's serum so we will use this as a working example:

- A plate containing the antigen for the antibody being tested is exposed to the patient's serum; any of the appropriate antibody present in the serum will bind the antigen on the plate.
- The enzyme used to catalyse the production of the coloured product (which is covalently attached to an antibody that is specific for the Fc portion of the antibody in the patient's serum) is added (see Fig. 12.24).
- The enzyme substrate is then added and the colour conversion occurs.

Each of these steps is incubated for a consistent period of time with any excess being washed before the next substance is added.

In addition to the ELISA test we can detect antibody by agglutination, for example:

- Coombs test
- Rheumatoid factor.

Flow cytometry and immunofluorescence

Flow cytometry is a useful tool for differentiating between different populations of cells, as well as for counting the number of cells within a sample. This is done by

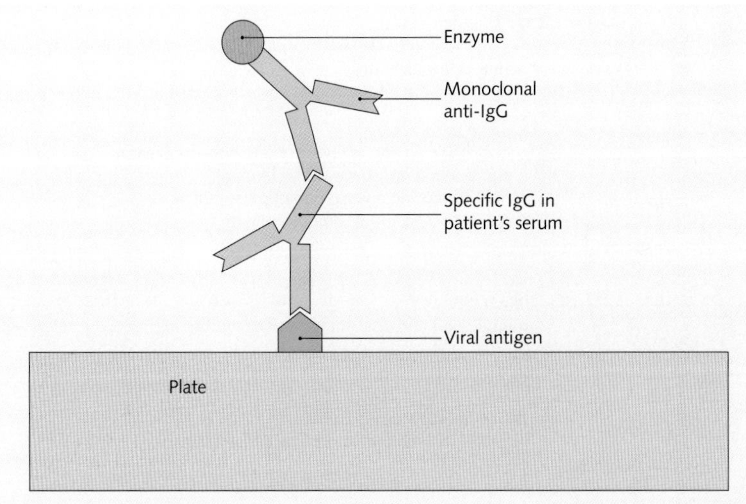

Fig. 12.24 Enzyme-linked immunosorbent assay (ELISA). ELISA can be used to detect antigens but is most commonly used to measure antibody to specific antigen (e.g. a virus) and this is shown. Viral antigen is bound to a plate and the patient's serum added. If specific IgG is present it will bind to the antigen. Enzyme labelled anti-IgG is added (binding to the patient's IgG). The enzyme converts a colourless substrate into a coloured product. The intensity of colour is relative to the amount of antigen.

producing a very fine stream of cells in suspension, where only one cell at a time passes through a beam of laser light. Sensors detect when a cell blocks the beam of light and the amount of light scatter identifies the size and granularity of the cell. Various surface antigens on the cell can be bound by monoclonal antibodies (specific for one antigen). The monoclonal antibodies are labelled with dyes that fluoresce under laser light (immunofluorescence). Different types of dye allow the detection of specific antigens (most machines use red and green fluorescence, but up to five colours are used by some machines); CD4 counts (T cell counts) are done in this way.

Medical intervention

Objectives

You should be able to:

- Understand the concepts of immunization
- Understand the process of organ transplantation and precautions taken to prevent rejection
- Explain the mechanisms of drugs used to suppress the immune system and reduce inflammation.

IMMUNIZATION

Concepts of immunization

HINTS AND TIPS

It is important to be able to explain the difference between active and passive immunity. Active immunity is an immune response (conferring immunological memory) produced by the body in response to antigen (either infection or vaccination). Passive immunity, however, is the temporary immunity that occurs when preformed antibodies are passed to an individual.

Immunity can be achieved by passive or active immunization (Fig. 13.1).

Passive immunization

This is a temporary immunity that results from the transfer of exogenous antibody and thus occurs without prior exposure to the specific antigens. Passive immunity is seen in the fetus when maternal IgG crosses the placenta and in breast-fed babies due to the IgA content of breast milk. Passive immunity can be conferred to individuals exposed to a pathogen to which they are not immune by the injection of immunoglobulins to the antigen. These are taken from blood donors immune to the pathogen, e.g. a non-immunized patient exposed to hepatitis B would benefit from this kind of post-infection prophylaxis.

HINTS AND TIPS

Examples where passive immunity is used:
- Prevent hepatitis A and B infection
- Prevent varicella zoster
- Treat snake bites (anti-venom).

Active immunization

Active immunization results from contact with antigens, either through natural infection or by vaccination. Individuals exhibit a primary immune response, with clonal expansion of B and T cells and formation of memory cells. Subsequent exposure to the same antigen will induce a secondary immune response (see Chapter 10).

Vaccination

Vaccination is a form of active immunization that induces specific immunity to a particular pathogen. The aim is to produce a rapid, protective immune response on re-exposure to that pathogen. An ideal vaccine is:

- Safe, with minimal side-effects and free from contaminating substances
- Immunogenic, activating the required branches of the immune system, inducing long-lasting local and systemic immunity
- Heat stable, because there are difficulties with refrigeration, particularly in tropical countries
- Inexpensive, an important consideration, especially in developing countries.

Types of vaccine

The types of vaccine in current use are listed in Figure 13.2. Vaccines are live attenuated (weakened) organisms, killed organisms or subunit; the features of each are compared in Figure 13.3. The routine immunization schedule used in the UK is shown in Figure 13.4.

HINTS AND TIPS

A healthy immune system can cope with live attenuated vaccines. However, they should never be given to immunocompromised patients as they can cause severe infection.

Fig. 13.1 Comparison of passive and active immunity

	Passive	**Active**
Features	Preformed immunoglobulins transferred to individual Large amounts of antibody available immediately Short lifespan of antibodies	Contact with antigen induces adaptive immune response Takes some time to develop immunity Long-lived immunity induced – includes T cells, B cells and antibody
Examples	Antitetanus toxin antibody	Natural exposure; vaccination

Fig. 13.2 Different types of vaccine in use in the UK today

Vaccine	**Features**	**Examples**
Live attenuated	Attenuation achieved by repeated culture on artificial media or by serial passage in animals; immunogenicity is retained, but virulence is significantly diminished	Oral polio (Sabin), BCG, measles, mumps, rubella (MMR)
Killed	Intact organisms killed by exposure to heat or chemicals, e.g. formalin	Intramuscular polio (Salk), pertussis, influenza
Subunit	Purified, protective immunity-inducing antigenic components; often surface antigens	Non-conjugated pneumococcal, acellular pertussis
Recombinant	Genes encoding epitopes, which elicit protective immunity, are inserted into pro- or eukaryotic cells; large quantities of vaccine are produced rapidly	Hepatitis B surface antigen (produced in yeast cells), human papilloma virus (HPV) vaccines
Toxoids	Bacterial toxins inactivated by heat or chemicals	Diphtheria, tetanus
Conjugates	Polysaccharide antigen is linked to protein carrier to enhance immunogenicity	*Haemophilus influenzae* type B (Hib), meningococcal, pneumococcal

BCG, bacille Calmette–Guérin.

Fig. 13.3 Features of live versus killed vaccines

Feature	**Live attenuated vaccine**	**Killed vaccine**
Level of immunity induced	High: organism replicates at site of infection (mimicking natural infection)	Low: non-replicating organisms produce a short-lived stimulus
Cell-mediated response	Good: antigens are processed and presented with MHC molecules	Poor
Local immunity	Good	Poor
Cost	Expensive to produce and administer	Cheaper than live vaccines
Reversion to virulence	Possible but rare	No (therefore safe for immunocompromised and pregnant patients)
Stability	Heat labile	Heat stable
Risk of contamination	Possible, e.g. by virus in cell media	N/A

The genes of attenuated organisms can differ from the wild type by just a few base pairs. It is relatively easy for them to mutate back to the disease-causing strain. MHC, major histocompatibility complex; N/A, not applicable.

Fig. 13.4 Routine immunization schedule used in the UK

Age	Vaccine
Neonate (only high-risk groups)	BCG
2 months (2 injections)	Diphtheria, tetanus, (acellular) pertussis, polio and *Haemophilus influenzae* type b (DTaP/IPV/Hib). Known as the 5-in-1. Pneumococcal conjugate vaccine (PCV)
3 months (2 injections)	DTaP/IPV/Hib Meningococcal type C (MenC)
4 months (3 injections)	DTaP/IPV/Hib PVC MenC
12–13 months (3 injections)	MMR PVC Hib/MenC
3 years 4 months −5 years (2 injections)	DTaP/IPV MMR
12–13 years (girls only)	Human papillomavirus (HPV) types 16 and 18
13–18 years (1 injection)	DT/IPV
Adult	Boosters for tetanus and polio
> 65 years	Annual influenza Pneumococcal polysaccharide vaccine (PPV). One-off
Any age	Occupation, e.g. Hep A, Hep B Travel, e.g. Yellow fever

Vaccines are not 100% efficacious. A small proportion of individuals receiving vaccination will not respond adequately. However, by immunizing the majority of the population, non-responders are unlikely to come into contact with the virus because the viral reservoir is reduced (herd immunity).

Vaccination against toxins such as tetanus does not provide immunity against the toxin-producing bacterium (*Clostridium tetani*). Its benefits come from preventing the sequelae associated with the tetanus toxin, i.e. tetanus of the masseter muscles (lock jaw).

You will notice that a number of vaccinations are given simultaneously; this is not just for convenience. Given alone some of the subunit vaccines would not evoke a sufficient immune response in order for immunity to develop. For example, the DTaP vaccination relies strongly on the danger signal produced in response to the killed pertussis organism to develop immunity to the diphtheria and tetanus toxoids.

HINTS AND TIPS

It is possible to enhance the immune response to vaccines by using adjuvants. Adjuvants, e.g. aluminium salts and *Bordetella pertussis*, are non-specific stimulators of the pattern recognition molecules of the innate immune system. When these are present, the innate immune system transmits a 'danger signal' to the adaptive immune system to promote a good response.

TRANSPLANTATION

Mechanisms of solid organ transplant rejection

Autologous grafts are grafts moved from one part of the body to another, e.g. skin grafts.
Syngeneic grafts are between genetically identical individuals, e.g. monozygotic twins.
Allogeneic grafts are between individuals of the same species.
Xenogeneic grafts are between different species.

Unless the donor and recipient are immunologically identical, the recipient will mount a rejection response against 'foreign' antigens expressed by the graft. The most important graft antigens responsible for an immune response in the recipient are the major histocompatibility complex (MHC) molecules (see p. 92). However, even when the donor and recipient are genetically identical at the MHC loci, graft rejection can occur due to differences at other loci, which encode minor histocompatibility antigens. A rejection response can lead to loss of a graft. There are three types of graft rejection (Fig. 13.5):

1. Hyperacute: occurs within hours as a result of preformed antibodies, type II hypersensitivity reaction
2. Acute: takes several days to develop, type IV hypersensitivity reaction
3. Chronic: occurs months to years after transplantation; can be caused by a variety of mechanisms. It cannot be treated.

Fig. 13.5 Patterns of graft rejection

Type	Mechanism	Prevention
Hyperacute (minutes–hours)	Pre-existing antidonor antibodies	Perform cross-match of donor cells and recipient's serum, check for ABO compatibility
Acute (days–weeks)	T cell mediated	HLA matching of donor and recipient, antirejection therapy
Chronic (months–years)	Unclear	HLA matching

HLA, human leucocyte antigen.

Fig. 13.6 Common transplants

Transplant	Notes
Kidney	Live or cadaveric donor; the fewer the MHC mismatches, the greater the success rate; must be ABO compatible
Heart	Matching is beneficial, but often time is a more pressing concern
Liver	No evidence to suggest that matching affects graft survival; rejection less aggressive than for other organs
Skin graft	Most grafts are autologous, but allografts can be used to protect burns patients
Corneal graft	Matching (class II MHC) is required only if a previous graft was vascularized
Stem cell	Host-versus-graft (HVG) or graft-versus-host (GVH) responses possible. The transplant must be well matched and antirejection therapy used. Host immune cells are destroyed by irradiation prior to transplant (avoids HVG). T cells are depleted from the graft (avoids GVH) using monoclonal antibody and complement

MHC, major histocompatibility complex.

Strategies for preventing rejection

Human leucocyte antigen (HLA) typing and antibody cross-matching

The ideal match is that between monozygotic twins. In all other situations there will be some genetic disparity between donor and recipient. The aim of matching is to minimize genetic differences between donor and recipient. Both the donor and recipient will be HLA typed.

Antirejection therapy

Immunosuppressive drugs can be used to prevent rejection by suppressing antibody and T cell responses. Examples of drugs used include:

- Steroids: these are anti-inflammatory (see below)
- Azathioprine, mycophenolate mofetil and methotrexate: antiproliferative drugs
- Tacrolimus, ciclosporin and rapamycin: inhibit signalling in T cells.

The disadvantage of such non-specific therapy is that the recipient is at increased risk of opportunistic infections (e.g. cytomegalovirus) and certain malignancies. Most transplant patients will stay on these drugs for life as rejection can still take place many years after transplantation.

Newer, more selective agents are being developed, including anti-CD3 and anti-IL-2 receptor monoclonal antibodies. IL-2 receptor monoclonal antibodies block the growth factor needed by all types of lymphocyte. Thus, they are very potent immunosuppressants and are only used to treat rejection rather than prevent it.

Common types of transplantation performed today are summarized in Fig. 13.6.

Stem cell transplant

Stem cell transplants are used in the treatment of some cancers and primary immunodeficiencies. Stem cells are obtained from bone marrow or blood. Imperfectly matched stem cells can be rejected by the recipient. In addition, stem cells give rise to lymphocytes, which can attack the host, causing acute or chronic graft-versus-host disease.

ANTI-INFLAMMATORY DRUGS

Anti-inflammatory drugs are used commonly for the treatment of a variety of hypersensitivity reactions. Different types of anti-inflammatory drug are available, including:

- Corticosteroids
- Non-steroidal anti-inflammatory drugs
- Other anti-inflammatory agents.

Corticosteroids

The adrenal cortex releases several steroid hormones into the circulation. Glucocorticoids not only affect carbohydrate and protein metabolism, but also have effects on the immune system, acting as immunosuppressive and anti-inflammatory agents. Several glucocorticoids are available therapeutically, including:

- Hydrocortisone: can be given intravenously in status asthmaticus or topically for inflammatory skin conditions
- Prednisolone: oral preparations are given in many inflammatory or allergic conditions
- Beclometasone: used as an aerosol in asthma or topically for eczema.

Conditions commonly treated with steroids include:

- Inflammatory bowel disease
- Allergic conditions, e.g. asthma
- Severe inflammatory skin conditions
- Severe inflammatory rheumatological conditions.

Corticosteroids work primarily on phagocytes. They inhibit the production of mediators of inflammation (prostaglandins, cytokines) and prevent antigen presentation. At high doses they have direct effects on lymphocytes.

Adverse effects and contraindications

Glucocorticoids cause many adverse effects at the high doses required to produce an anti-inflammatory effect. Glucocorticoids can cause hundreds of adverse effects, and many patients find them too much to put up with. The clinical features are similar to those seen in Cushing's syndrome and some important adverse effects are shown in Figure 13.7.

Fig. 13.7 Some adverse effects of glucocorticoids and their prevention or treatment

Adverse effect	Prevention or treatment
Diabetes	Regular blood sugar measurements
Osteoporosis	Bone density should be regularly monitored during steroid treatment. Patients, especially the elderly, may need bisphosphonates and calcium supplements
Peptic ulcer	Proton pump inhibitors may be required
Thin skin, easy bruising and poor wound healing	No treatment, but early and intensive intervention of wounds is necessary to prevent chronic morbidity
Adrenal insufficiency	Prevent sudden decreases in dose, increase dose when ill and carry a steroid card. Treatment is with resuscitation and steroid replacement

Steroids are contraindicated if there is evidence of systemic infection. Long-term high-dose steroid therapy is usually avoided. When they are used long term, there should be regular checks on blood pressure, blood sugar and bone density. Care should be taken when reducing a dose of steroids. The adrenal cortex requires time to recover so sharp reductions in dose can result in an adrenal (Adisonian) crisis.

Non-steroidal anti-inflammatory drugs (NSAIDs)

NSAIDs include a large number of drugs that can be bought over the counter, e.g. aspirin, ibuprofen, diclofenac. They are chemically diverse but all act to inhibit cyclo-oxygenase (Fig. 13.8). This attenuates, but does not abolish, inflammation. As well as their anti-inflammatory effects, NSAIDs have analgesic and antipyretic actions. They are used primarily in conditions where pain is accompanied by inflammation, such as rheumatoid arthritis.

Cyclo-oxygenase (COX) mainly occurs as two isoenzymes: COX-1 and COX-2. COX-1 is responsible for the physiological prostaglandins that protect the gastric mucosa, prevent platelet aggregation and protect renal function. COX-2 is important for the formation of proinflammatory prostaglandins. Thus the important side-effects of NSAIDs, including peptic ulcers and renal failure, occur mainly as a result of COX-1 inhibition. Most NSAIDs block both COX isoenzymes, but some are more active against one or the other. Selective COX-2 inhibitors (e.g. celecoxib) were released in the hope of having anti-inflammatory effects without gastric and renal side-effects; however, they were withdrawn from the market due to an increased incidence of cardio- and cerebrovascular events.

Aspirin

Acetylsalicylic acid (aspirin) is anti-inflammatory but causes a lot of adverse effects. As a consequence of this, newer NSAIDs (e.g. ibuprofen) are usually preferred for treatment of inflammatory conditions, because they exhibit fewer side-effects. Aspirin is far more efficient at inhibiting COX-1 (hence the side-effects) and is used prophylactically in low doses in people who have had strokes or have ischaemic heart disease because of its ability to inhibit platelet function (see p. 59).

Paracetamol

Paracetamol has good analgesic and antipyretic properties but little effect on inflammation. Thus it is not strictly an NSAID but is usually grouped with them for ease.

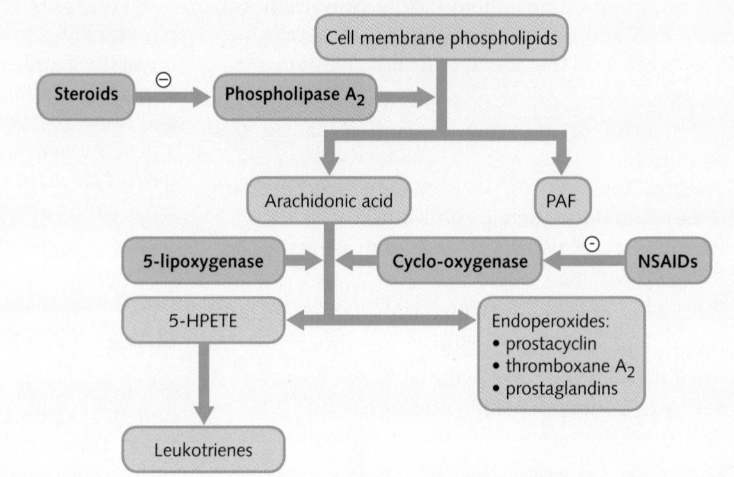

Fig. 13.8 The actions of non-steroidal anti-inflammatory drugs (NSAIDs) in arachidonic acid metabolism. COX, cyclo-oxygenase.

Adverse effects and contraindications

Adverse effects with NSAIDs are common. They often cause damage to the mucosa of the gastrointestinal tract because they remove the cytoprotective effects of prostaglandins in the gut; the mucosa becomes ulcerated because of the damaging effects of stomach acid. Many NSAID preparations, e.g. enteric-coating, are designed to reduce ulceration. NSAIDs can also be nephrotoxic and cause bronchospasm. Side-effects of aspirin include nausea, vomiting, epigastric pain and tinnitus.

Other anti-inflammatory drugs

Other anti-inflammatory drugs reduce inflammation via different mechanisms. These include:

- Immunosuppressive drugs, such as ciclosporin and azathioprine (main effects on T cells)
- Methotrexate (main effects on macrophages).

Such drugs are often used in chronic inflammatory conditions, e.g. rheumatoid arthritis, to reduce the need for steroids. Each drug has specific adverse effects and contraindications. Newer approaches use biological agents to block the effects of proinflammatory cytokines. For example, the effects of TNF can be blocked by infliximab (monoclonal anti-TNF) or etanercept (soluble TNF receptor). Both drugs are very effective in the treatment of rheumatoid arthritis and Crohn's disease. However, they can increase the risk of infections, such as tuberculosis, in which TNF normally has a protective role.

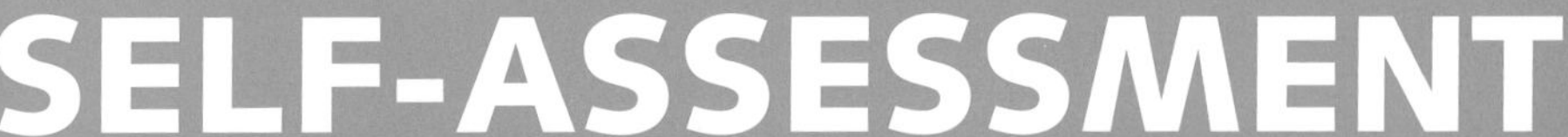

SELF-ASSESSMENT

Multiple Choice Questions (MCQs)

1. Which **one** of the following answers corresponds with where haemopoiesis is primarily situated in a fetus, at 3 months gestation?
   a. Marrow of all bones.
   b. Liver and spleen.
   c. Fetal yolk sac.
   d. Marrow of axial skeleton.
   e. Lymph nodes.

2. Lymphoid progenitor cells travel to which organ to become T lymphocytes?
   a. Spleen.
   b. Liver.
   c. Thymus.
   d. Kidney.
   e. Thyroid.

3. A 65-year-old patient receiving chemotherapy for a disseminated malignancy attends hospital with signs of an infection. A full blood count reveals that he has a neutrophil count of $< 0.1 \times 10^9$/L (normal range 2.0–7.5 $\times$ 10^9/L). Which haemopoietic growth factor would help improve his neutrophil count?
   a. G-CSF.
   b. EPO.
   c. Romiplostim.
   d. Eltrombopag.
   e. Stem cell factor.

4. A patient suffering with idiopathic thrombocytopenic purpura undergoes a splenectomy. She is advised to get the pneumococcal vaccine booster every 5–10 years. Which of the following properties of *Strep. pneumoniae* make her prone to infection by this organism?
   a. It is gram positive.
   b. It is α-haemolytic.
   c. It is encapsulated.
   d. It causes pneumonia.
   e. It is a diplococcus.

5. Concerning bone marrow in the adult, which **one** of the following is correct?
   a. It is the only tissue in the body capable of haemopoiesis .
   b. Yellow marrow is where haemopoiesis normally takes place.
   c. It contains neutrophils which store iron for the developing erythrocyte.
   d. Red marrow is normally restricted to the axial skeleton and the proximal ends of long bones.
   e. It contains red and yellow marrow, as well as red and white pulps.

6. Regarding erythrocytes, which **one** of the following is correct?
   a. They have a bilobed nucleus.
   b. They are derived from lymphoid progenitor cells.
   c. They transport CO_2.
   d. They have an average lifespan of 12 days.
   e. They have a spherical shape.

7. Concerning iron metabolism, which **one** of the following is correct?
   a. Iron is absorbed in the stomach.
   b. Excess iron is readily excreted.
   c. Iron is transported in the blood bound to apoferritin.
   d. Primary haemochromatosis is caused by excessive iron absorption.
   e. Total body stores of iron are 4 mg.

8. Concerning haemoglobin, which **one** of the following is correct?
   a. Adult haemoglobin contains 4 identical globin chains.
   b. Each haemoglobin can carry 4 molecules of oxygen.
   c. Oxygen binding follows a hyperbolic curve.
   d. 2,3-diphosphoglycerate levels rise in hypoxia to allow increased oxygen uptake by haemoglobin.
   e. The Bohr effect (a shift of the oxygen dissociation curve to the right) is due to decreased H^+ concentration.

9. Concerning fetal haemoglobin, which **one** of the following is correct?
   a. It may be raised in β-thalassaemia syndromes.
   b. It is composed of two α- and two β-globin chains.
   c. It has a lower affinity for oxygen than adult haemoglobin.
   d. It remains the primary haemoglobin in infants until approximately 2 years of age.
   e. It is normally about 2% of the haemoglobin in adults.

10. Regarding haem production and metabolism, which **one** of the following is correct?
    a. Haem is produced in mitochondria in the liver.
    b. Haem is broken down by macrophages in the gut.
    c. Haem consists of four Fe^{2+} ions and a protoporphyrin ring.
    d. Conjugated bilirubin is secreted into lymph.
    e. Unconjugated bilirubin is water insoluble.

11. Concerning erythropoietin (EPO), which **one** of the following is correct?
    a. It is a steroid hormone.

b. It is mainly secreted by the Kupffer cells and hepatocytes in the liver.
c. The major stimulus for secretion is higher androgen levels.
d. Blood levels of EPO are raised at higher altitudes.
e. Splenectomy reduces levels of EPO, resulting in anaemia.

12. Concerning vitamin B_{12}, which **one** of the following is correct?
a. It is absorbed in the proximal jejunum.
b. It requires extrinsic factor for absorption.
c. It can also be synthesized by the skin.
d. It is stored in the bone marrow.
e. Total gastrectomy reduces absorption.

13. Regarding folic acid, which **one** of the following is correct?
a. Pernicious anaemia is a common cause of folic acid deficiency.
b. It is exclusively found in animal products.
c. It is utilized in the metabolism of alcohol.
d. It is absorbed in the stomach.
e. Folic acid deficiency requires an injection every 3 months.

14. A normochromic, normocytic anaemia is most commonly associated with which **one** of the following?
a. Iron deficiency.
b. Renal failure.
c. Pernicious anaemia.
d. Thalassaemia.
e. Hereditary spherocytosis.

15. Which **one** of the following is a feature of iron deficiency anaemia?
a. Leuconychia.
b. Macrocytic, hypochromic red cells.
c. Raised serum ferritin.
d. Raised serum transferrin.
e. Subacute combined degeneration of the cord.

16. A 70-year-old woman presents to her GP with tiredness and dizzy-spells. Which **one** of the following blood results would most favour a diagnosis of anaemia of chronic disease, rather than iron deficiency anaemia?
a. Haemoglobin 8.5 g/dL.
b. Mean corpuscular volume (MCV) 75 fL.
c. Low serum iron.
d. Low total iron-binding capacity (TIBC).
e. Negative direct Coombs test.

17. Which **one** of the following is a feature of haemolytic anaemia?
a. Cholesterol gallstones.
b. Raised serum haptoglobin.
c. Glossitis.
d. Jaundice.
e. Splenic atrophy.

18. Which **one** of the following is a common side effect of oral iron supplementation?
a. Angina.
b. Peripheral neuropathy.
c. Constipation.
d. Brittle, spoon shaped nails (koilonychia).
e. Mouth ulcers.

19. A 62-year-old male, with no past medical history of note, presents with fatigue. On examination there is pallor of the mucous membranes, as well as angular stomatitis. A full blood count revealed the following results: Hb 9.5 g/dL (normal range for men 13–17 g/dL) and mean corpuscular volume (MCV) 69 fL (normal range 80–100 fL). Iron studies reveal a low serum iron, a low serum ferritin and a high total iron-binding capacity (TIBC). Which **one** of the following is the most appropriate next investigation?
a. Plasma electrophoresis.
b. Endoscopy of the gastrointestinal tract.
c. Clotting tests.
d. Urinalysis.
e. Trephine bone marrow biopsy.

20. Which of the following statements is true of haemochromatosis?
a. Clinical features normally present in the teens.
b. It is associated with mutations in the phosphatidylinositol glycan protein A (PIG-A) gene.
c. Iron deficiency anaemia is a common complication.
d. Inheritance is autosomal dominant.
e. Diabetes mellitus is a common complication.

21. A 44-year-old woman presents for the first time to his GP. She complains of fatigue. On examination she is pale, and looks dishevelled. Full blood count reveals the following blood results: Hb 10 g/dL (normal range for women 12–15 g/dL), mean corpuscular volume (MCV) 102 fL (normal range 80–100 fL). The GP calls the patient back to take some blood for iron studies, as well as vitamin B_{12} and folate levels. Again she is dishevelled, and this time smells of alcohol at 11.15 a.m. Which **one** of the following results do you most expect to see?
a. Low serum iron.
b. Low serum folate.
c. High total iron-binding capacity.
d. Low serum vitamin B_{12}.
e. Low ferritin.

22. A 32-year-old woman is diagnosed with a megaloblastic anaemia. Autoantibodies against intrinsic factor and gastric parietal cells are positive. Before commencement of vitamin B_{12} replacement

which of the following precautions is the most important?
a. Measure initial vitamin B_{12}.
b. Do a pregnancy test.
c. Check that she is not allergic to vitamin B_{12}.
d. Check that she doesn't have swallowing difficulties.
e. Measure serum folate.

23. Approximately how often are vitamin B_{12} injections administered to patients with vitamin B_{12} deficiency?
a. Every week.
b. Every 4 weeks.
c. Every 3 months.
d. Every year.
e. Every 3 years.

24. A newborn, Caucasian boy is noticed to be jaundiced. Full blood count reveals a macrocytic anaemia. The boy's mother says that she thinks his estranged father had a splenectomy. A peripheral blood film is performed and his red cells appear smaller and thicker than normal. Which of the following is the most likely diagnosis?
a. Glucose-6-phosphate dehydrogenase deficiency.
b. Sickle cell anaemia.
c. Pyruvate kinase deficiency.
d. Hereditary spherocytosis.
e. B-thalassaemia major.

25. Which of the following features would suggest β-thalassaemia minor, as opposed to β-thalassaemia major?
a. Onset of symptoms at 9 months of age.
b. Full blood count showing a severe microcytic, hypochromic anaemia.
c. Skull X-ray showing 'hair-on-end' appearance.
d. The presence of HbA on electrophoresis.
e. Splenomegaly.

26. Which **one** of the following statements about lymphocytes is correct?
a. They are usually larger than other white cells.
b. Their nucleus is small to allow more granules.
c. They spend most of their time circulating in the blood.
d. They come from myeloid stem cells.
e. B cells and natural killer (NK) cells tend to be bigger than T cells.

27. Which **one** of the following statements about neutrophils is correct?
a. Left shift means that the nuclei are hypersegmented.
b. They normally have one large, circular nucleus.
c. Primarily respond to parasitic infections.
d. Immature 'band' forms may appear in severe sepsis.
e. They make up a small proportion of the circulating white cells.

28. Which **one** of the following white blood cells is the least common white cell in the blood and is functionally very similar to mast cells?
a. Neutrophils.
b. Basophils.
c. Eosinophils.
d. Monocytes.
e. Lymphoctyes.

29. Which of the following statements describes myelodysplastic syndromes?
a. Bone marrow disorders resulting in excess of one or more type of myeloid cell.
b. Bone marrow disorders that result in the clonal production of abnormal myeloid cells.
c. A collection of diseases that result in a clonal proliferation of white blood cells.
d. Clonal proliferations of lymphoid cells, mainly from lymph nodes and extranodal tissue.
e. Malignant proliferation of plasma cells.

30. The Philadelphia chromosome is associated most heavily with which malignancy?
a. Hodgkin's lymphoma.
b. Acute myeloid leukaemia.
c. Chronic lymphoid leukaemia.
d. Chronic myeloid leukaemia.
e. Myeloma.

31. Bence-Jones protein is seen in which malignancy?
a. Hodgkin's lymphoma.
b. Non-Hodgkin's lymphoma.
c. Chronic myeloid leukaemia.
d. Chronic lymphocytic leukaemia.
e. Myeloma.

32. A 3-year-old boy presented to his GP with a persistent cough. Examination revealed bruising and splenomegaly. A full blood count showed that he was very anaemic and his white blood cells were markedly raised. Which **one** of the following is the **most likely** diagnosis?
a. Non-accidental injury.
b. Viral upper respiratory tract infection.
c. Acute lymphoblastic leukaemia.
d. Hodgkin's lymphoma.
e. Haemophilia A.

33. A 7-year-old boy from the Uganda presented to his GP with a 2-week history of jaw pain, fatigue, fever and sweating. Examination revealed a jaw mass. What is the **most likely** diagnosis?
a. β-thalassaemia major.
b. Acute lymphoblastic leukaemia.
c. Burkitt's lymphoma.
d. Sickle cell anaemia.
e. Acute myleloid leukaemia.

34. A 21-year-old university student presents to his GP with a painless swelling in his neck. He also reports

night sweats and weight loss. On examination his posterior cervical lymph nodes feel matted and rubbery. What abnormality would you most likely see in this patient?
a. A pepper-pot skull.
b. The Philadelphia chromosome.
c. Positive monospot test.
d. Reed-Sternberg cells.
e. The presence of more than 20% blast cells in the marrow.

35. Venesection is the treatment of choice for which **one** of the following disorders?
a. Primary polycythaemia.
b. Primary thrombocythaemia.
c. Myelofibrosis.
d. Acute myeloid leukaemia.
e. Non-Hodgkin's lymphoma.

36. With which **one** of the following tests could you observe the bone marrow architecture and cellularity?
a. Cytogenic analysis.
b. Lymph node biopsy.
c. Peripheral blood film.
d. Trephine biopsy.
e. Bone marrow aspirate.

37. Which **one** of the following statements about haemophilia A is correct?
a. Inheritance is autosomal dominant.
b. Prevalence depends on social class.
c. It is associated with pathological arthrodesis.
d. It is caused by a deficiency of factor IX.
e. A common feature is epistaxis.

38. Regards the haemostatic system, which of the following is true?
a. The FIXa-FVIIIa-Ca^{2+} complex converts prothrombin to thrombin.
b. The coagulation cascade culminates in thrombin cleaving fibrinogen into fibrin.
c. The activated partial thromboplastin time (APTT) assesses the extrinsic pathway.
d. Platelets are only involved in primary haemostasis.
e. Protein S inhibits FIIa and FVIIa.

39. Which of the following will prolong the prothrombin time?
a. von Willebrand's disease.
b. Haemophilia A.
c. Haemophilia B.
d. Protein C deficiency.
e. Warfarin therapy.

40. Which of the following statements regarding warfarin therapy is correct?
a. The lower the international normalised ratio (INR), the lower the risk of clotting.
b. Warfarin has a half-life of 20 hours.
c. Warfarin is teratogenic.
d. Warfarin mediates its effects mainly on the intrinsic pathway.
e. Warfarin is rarely affected by other medications.

41. How does aspirin mediate its anti-platelet effect?
a. It blocks the ADP receptor on the platelet surface.
b. It irreversibly inhibits cyclo-oxygenase.
c. It is a phosphodiesterase inhibitor.
d. It is a GPIIb/IIIa inhibitor.
e. It is a vitamin K antagonist.

42. Which **one** of the following statements is most associated with increased risk of thrombosis?
a. Aspirin therapy.
b. Liver disease.
c. von Willebrand's disease.
d. Atrial fibrillation (AF).
e. Anorexia.

43. Which **one** of the following is a vitamin-K-dependent clotting factor?
a. Fibrinogen
b. Prothrombin
c. Clotting factor V
d. Clotting factor VIII
e. Clotting factor XII

44. Low-molecular-weight heparin (LMWH) is monitored during pregnancy and in renal failure using which test?
a. The prothrombin time.
b. The activated partial thromboplastin time (APTT).
c. The thrombin time.
d. The bleeding time.
e. Anti-Xa assay.

45. Which **one** of the following statements regarding the ABO antigen system is correct?
a. Blood group A is the most common in the UK.
b. People who are blood group AB have antibodies to both the A and B red cell antigens.
c. Anti-A and anti-B antibodies are usually IgG.
d. A couple who are both blood group O will only have group O children.
e. Group O plasma can be given to patients with all blood groups.

46. Which **one** of the following statements is true regarding rhesus (Rh) antigens?
a. All anti-D antibodies are IgG.
b. Most Caucasians are Rh D negative.
c. Rh negative individuals are born with anti-D antibodies.
d. The least immunogenic Rh antigen is the D antigen.
e. All children of parents who are Rh D positive will be Rh D positive.

47. Which **one** of the following statements regarding haemolytic disease of the newborn (HDN) is correct?
a. It usually occurs with the first child.
b. It will not occur if the mother is rhesus D positive.
c. Rhesus D incompatibility is normally due to IgM antibodies.
d. Anti-D antibody should be given to all rhesus D negative mothers during pregnancy.
e. It results in a mild anaemia due to haemolysis.

48. Which **one** of the following signs would raise most suspicion of an acute haemolytic transfusion reaction?
a. Cyanosis.
b. Severe hypertension.
c. Low back pain.
d. Hypothermia.
e. Bradycardia.

49. Massive transfusions can result in coagulopathies because packed red cells are deficient in clotting factors. The two clotting factors most deficient are factor V and which **one** other clotting factor?
a. Factor II.
b. Factor VII.
c. Factor VIII.
d. Factor IX.
e. Factor XII.

50. A 55-year-old woman undergoes a hysterectomy. During surgery her vena cava is damaged. She proceeds to lose a great deal of blood but the vena cava is eventually repaired. Over the course of the next 24 hours she receives 12 units of cross-matched red cells. She appears much better. The foundation doctor orders some clotting tests and notices that the prothrombin time (PT) and the activated partial thromboplastin time (APTT) are both prolonged. Which blood product should be given?
a. Albumin.
b. Fresh frozen plasma.
c. O negative red cells.
d. Whole blood.
e. Anti-D immunoglobulin.

51. Concerning the innate immune response, which **one** of the following is correct?
a. It is a specific response to a particular antigen.
b. The response improves with repeated exposure.
c. It is composed of phagocytes and complement.
d. It is good at combating intracellular pathogens.
e. It takes a long time to develop.

52. Concerning the adaptive immune system, which **one** of the following is correct?
a. CD8 positive T cells phagocytose cells.
b. T cells produce antibodies which enable other parts of the immune system to confront pathogens.
c. T helper cells are normally CD8 positive.
d. CD4 positive T lymphocytes recognise antigen associated with MHC class II.
e. The main function of plasma cells is to produce cytokines.

53. A pregnant patient asks her GP about the benefits of breast feeding. Which immunoglobulin is present in colostrum (early milk), and protects the mucosal surfaces of the intestines?
a. IgG.
b. IgM.
c. IgA.
d. IgD.
e. IgE.

54. Which **one** of the following is a phagocyte?
a. Macrophage.
b. Basophil.
c. B cell.
d. T cell.
e. The membrane attack complex.

55. During phagocytosis, the phagosome fuses with which **one** of the following organelles?
a. Nucleus.
b. Lysosome
c. Mitochondrion.
d. Golgi apparatus.
e. Endoplasmic reticulum.

56. Which **one** of the following types of cell are the major constituents in pus?
a. Plasma cells.
b. Macrophages.
c. Mast cells.
d. Eosinophils
e. Neutrophils.

57. Which **one** cell type can induce apoptosis of virally modified or cancerous cells?
a. Neutrophils.
b. Mast cells.
c. Eosinophils.
d. Natural killer cells.
e. B cells.

58. Which **one** of the following is an acute phase protein?
a. Tumour necrosis factor alpha.
b. C-reactive protein.
c. Interferon gamma.
d. Interleukin-1.
e. Transforming growth factor beta.

59. The classical pathway of the complement system is started by which processes?
a. Microbial surfaces, along with factor B and D, activate C3.
b. Antigen is presented by dendritic cells.
c. Mannan-binding lectin binds to some encapsulated bacteria.

d. Antigen-antibody complexes activate C1.
e. Class I MHC present intracellular antigen.

60. Which of the following complement factors or factor fragments are responsible for opsonization?
a. C3a.
b. C5b.
c. C5a
d. C3b.
e. C1.

61. The membrane attack complex mediates its actions on pathogens by which **one** of the following mechanisms?
a. Phagocytosis.
b. Opsonization.
c. Osmotic lysis.
d. It triggers apoptosis.
e. Degranulation.

62. Hereditary angioedema results from of which **one** of the following?
a. Mannan-binding lectin deficiency.
b. IgA deficiency.
c. C1 inhibitor deficiency.
d. Type I hypersensitivity.
e. Thymic aplasia.

63. Which **one** of the following statements about major histocompatability complex (MHC) is true?
a. Class II MHC presents endogenous antigens.
b. The haplotype is found on chromosome 6.
c. CD4 positive T cells bind class I MHC.
d. Class I MHC is only present on antigen-presenting cells.
e. Class I MHC presents peptides that are usually longer than class II MHC.

64. What is the name of the process whereby a B cell can produce different types of immunoglobulin, with the same specificity?
a. Junctional diversity.
b. Somatic hypermutation.
c. Affinity maturation.
d. Positive selection.
e. Class switching.

65. Which antibody is a pentamer?
a. IgM.
b. IgG.
c. IgA.
d. IgE.
e. IgD.

66. Regarding B cell activation, which **one** of the following statements is correct?
a. B cells are activated in the follicles of primary lymphoid organs.
b. The expression of bcl-2 results in apoptosis.
c. Somatic hypermutation of immunoglobulin genes occurs in the germinal centres.
d. B cells are activated following the presentation of antigen by neutrophils.
e. B cells are able to be activated and produce antibody without help from T cells.

67. Which antibody is important in the antiparasitic response?
a. IgG.
b. IgD.
c. IgM.
d. IgE.
e. IgA.

68. Which immunoglobulin is the main immunoglobulin in the secondary immune response?
a. IgG.
b. IgE.
c. IgD
d. IgA.
e. IgM.

69. Regarding the thymus, which **one** of the following statements is correct?
a. The embryonic thymus develops from the second pharyngeal pouch.
b. It begins to reduce in size after puberty.
c. It has four lobes.
d. It is located in the anterior mediastinum.
e. Most of the thymocytes in the thymus will mature and leave the thymus via the cortex.

70. The autosomal dominant condition that is caused by a deletion on chromosome 22, and resulting in thymic aplasia is which **one** of the following?
a. Down syndrome.
b. Edwards' syndrome.
c. DiGeorge syndrome.
d. Patau's syndrome.
e. Graves' disease.

71. Which **one** of the following is an example of a T cell superantigen, capable of causing toxic shock syndrome?
a. Nickel.
b. Staphylococcal enterotoxin.
c. Rheumatoid factor.
d. Acellular pertussis.
e. Bacille Calmette–Guerin

72. With regards acute inflammation, which **one** of the following processes normally occurs?
a. Local vasoconstriction.
b. Decreased vascular permeability.
c. Homing due to integrin molecules.
d. Leucocytes leave the tissues.
e. Inhibition of histamine.

73. Which **one** of the following is an example of mucosal-associated lymphoid tissue (MALT)?
a. Thymus.
b. Inguinal lymph nodes.
c. Bone marrow.
d. Peyer's patches.
e. Thyroid.

74. Concerning IgG immunoglobulin, which one of the following statements is true?
a. There are four Fab fragments.
b. There are two Fc fragments.
c. The amino terminal (N) domain of the light chain is constant.
d. The heavy chain determines the class of immunoglobulin.
e. The domain at the carboxyl (C) terminal of the light chain is variable.

75. Regarding the immune response to viruses, which **one** of the following is true?
a. Antibodies can neutralize virus particles, as well as act as an opsonin against virally infected cells.
b. Interferon gamma acts on neighbouring cells by inhibiting transcription and translation of viral proteins.
c. Viral peptides are presented on class II MHC molecules.
d. CD4 positive T cells are able to destroy infected cells.
e. CD8 positive T cells help antibody production, as well as the recruitment and activation of macrophages.

76. Varicella zoster evades the immune system by which **one** of the following mechanisms:
a. Being a latent virus.
b. Antigenic shift and drift.
c. Polymorphism.
d. Infection of lymphocytes.
e. Modulation of MHC expression.

77. Which one of the following components of the immune system can prevent bacterial pathogens present at a mucosal surface from entering the body?
a. Lysozyme.
b. C3b.
c. Neutrophils.
d. Dendritic cells.
e. Secretory immunoglobulin A (sIgA).

78. Which characteristic of Gram-negative bacteria makes them susceptible to the membrane attack complex (MAC)?
a. They are prokaryotic.
b. They have pili.
c. They have capsule of branched polysaccharides.
d. They have a lipid bilayer.
e. They have flagellae.

79. Most extracellular bacteria are killed by which immunological cells?
a. Cytotoxic CD8 positive T cells.
b. The membrane attack complex (MAC).
c. CD4 positive T helper cells.
d. Natural killer cells.
e. Phagocytes.

80. Which **one** of the following statements is true of protozoal infections?
a. Protozoa tend to cause extracellular infections.
b. Protozoa have complex life cycles which present the immune system with a variety of challenges.
c. Protozoa themselves cause significant damage to cells and tissues.
d. The immune system is efficient at dealing with protozoa, and infections are usually short-lived.
e. There are many protozoa that are pathogenic to humans.

81. Along with IgE and mast cells, which white blood cell is most important in combating parasitic worm infections?
a. Dendritic cells
b. Monocytes.
c. Neutrophils.
d. Eosinophils.
e. Lymphocytes.

82. Which type of immune dysfunction is characterized, in immunological terms, by IgE-mediated degranulation of mast cells?
a. Nickel allergy.
b. ABO incompatibility.
c. Allergic rhinitis.
d. Farmer's lung.
e. Rheumatoid arthritis.

83. Which one of the following investigations is most useful in type I hypersensitivity?
a. Skin prick testing.
b. Anti-double stranded DNA antibody assay.
c. Rheumatoid factor assay.
d. Patch testing.
e. C-reactive protein measurement.

84. Which one of the following is an example of type III hypersensitivity?
a. Eczema.
b. Farmer's lung.
c. Asthma.
d. Haemolytic disease of the newborn.
e. Nickel allergy.

85. Type IV hypersensitivity is mainly mediated by which cells?
a. Neutrophils.
b. Plasma cells.
c. CD8 positive T cells.
d. Mast cells.
e. T helper cells.

86. A 21-year-old man is brought to Accident and Emergency due to breathing problems that he developed after eating a sandwich in a local bakery. He has an audible stridor, is warm to the touch and has obvious facial oedema. Which one of the following is the most appropriate next step in his management?
- a. IV fluid challenge.
- b. Chloramphenamine IV.
- c. Hydrocortisone IV
- d. IM adrenaline (0.5 mL of 1:1000).
- e. C1 inhibitor IV.

87. Which of the following autoimmune diseases is caused by antibodies against the acetylcholine receptor?
- a. Coeliac disease.
- b. Graves' disease.
- c. Myasthenia gravis.
- d. Goodpasture's syndrome.
- e. Pernicious anaemia.

88. Antibodies against tissue transglutaminase are most associated with which of the following autoimmune conditions?
- a. Rheumatoid arthritis.
- b. Coeliac disease.
- c. Type I diabetes.
- d. Hashimoto's thyroiditis.
- e. Pernicious anaemia.

89. Which of the following is an example of an autoimmune disease caused by type IV hypersensitivity?
- a. Contact dermatitis.
- b. Rheumatoid arthritis.
- c. Systemic lupus erythematosus.
- d. Grave's disease.
- e. Farmer's lung.

90. Which one of the following cytokines is most involved in the pathogenesis of rheumatoid arthritis?
- a. Interleukin-8.
- b. Tumour necrosis factor alpha.
- c. Interleukin-17.
- d. Transforming growth factor beta.
- e. Interferon gamma.

91. Rheumatoid factor is normally which **one** of the following?
- a. IgM anti-IgG antibodies.
- b. IgA anti-IgM antibodies.
- c. IgE anti-IgG antibodies.
- d. IgD anti-IgE antibodies.
- e. IgG anti-IgM antibodies.

92. Which **one** of the following is a secondary immunodeficiency?
- a. DiGeorge syndrome.
- b. Chronic granulomatous disease.
- c. Acquired immunodeficiency syndrome.
- d. Wiskott–Aldrich syndrome.
- e. Severe combined immunodeficiency disease.

93. What type of virus is the human immunodeficiency virus (HIV)?
- a. A double-stranded DNA virus.
- b. A single-stranded DNA virus.
- c. A single-stranded RNA retrovirus.
- d. A double-stranded DNA retrovirus.
- e. A single-stranded RNA virus.

94. The human immunodeficiency virus (HIV) binds to the CD4 and CCR5 receptors via which **one** of the following proteins?
- a. p17.
- b. p24.
- c. p7.
- d. gp120.
- e. gp41.

95. Which of the following vaccines is a live attenuated vaccine?
- a. Diphtheria.
- b. Bacille Calmette–Guérin.
- c. Acellular pertussis.
- d. *Haemophilus influenzae* type B.
- e. Influenza.

96. Concerning vaccinations, which **one** of the following statements is correct?
- a. An ideal vaccine should not be immunogenic.
- b. The vaccines against measles, mumps and rubella (MMR) are recombinant vaccines.
- c. Killed vaccines are more expensive than live attenuated vaccines.
- d. Live attenuated vaccines produce a good cell-mediated response.
- e. Recombinant vaccines can rarely induce disease, especially in the immunocompromised.

97. Concerning transplant rejection, which **one** of the following statements is correct?
- a. Hyperacute rejection only occurs once the recipient has synthesized antibody to the graft.
- b. Acute cellular rejection is primarily mediated by natural killer cells.
- c. The mechanism of chronic rejection is well-understood and easy to treat.
- d. Hyperacute rejection is prevented by HLA-typing the donor organ and recipient.
- e. Acute cellular response takes several days to develop.

98. Which receptor is the target of newer anti-rejection therapies?
- a. Tumour necrosis factor alpha receptor.
- b. Transforming growth factor beta receptor.
- c. Interleukin-1 receptor.
- d. Interleukin-2 receptor.
- e. Interferon gamma receptor.

99. Which **one** of the following is a common adverse effect of non-steroidal anti-inflammatory drugs?
   a. Increased platelet aggregation.
   b. Gastritis.
   c. Cushing's syndrome.
   d. Osteoporosis.
   e. Fever.

100. Concerning the mechanism of non-steroidal anti-inflammatory drugs (NSAIDs), which **one** of the following statements is correct?
   a. NSAIDs act by inhibiting Phospholipase A_2.
   b. Hydrocortisone is often given orally for many inflammatory or allergic conditions.
   c. Paracetamol is one of the most potent anti-inflammatory drugs.
   d. Blockade of the cyclo-oxygenase 2 (COX-2) enzyme results in gastrointestinal side-effects.
   e. NSAIDs may be nephrotoxic and cause bronchospasm.

Extended Matching Questions (EMQs)

1. Concerning red blood cells:

A. Haemoglobin
B. Erythropoiesis
C. Bilirubin
D. Normoblasts
E. Erythropoietin (EPO)
F. Haemostasis
G. Transferrin
H. Erythrocyte
I. Reticulocyte
J. Haemopoietic stem cells

Instruction: For each scenario described below, choose the **single** most likely match from the above list of options. Each option may be used once, more than once, or not at all.

1. Highly glycosylated polypeptide hormone that stimulates the differentiation and maturation of erythrocytes.
2. Red blood cell component comprising two α-chains with either two β- or two δ-chains.
3. Breakdown product of red blood cells, which is conjugated in the liver and excreted in bile.
4. Immature red blood cells, present in the bone marrow, and in low numbers in the bloodstream.
5. Process by which red blood cells are made in the bone marrow.

2. Concerning the spleen and bone marrow:

A. Fetal yolk sac.
B. Fetal liver and spleen.
C. Red bone marrow.
D. Yellow bone marrow.
E. Haemopoietic islands.
F. Central longitudinal vein.
G. Red pulp of the spleen.
H. White pulp of the spleen.
I. Macrophages in the bone marrow.
J. Germinal centres of spleen.

Instruction: For each scenario described below, choose the **single** most likely match from the above list of options. Each option may be used once, more than once, or not at all.

1. Store iron in the form of ferritin and haemosiderin. This iron is used for haemopoiesis.
2. Type of bone marrow that is normally restricted to the axial skeleton and proximal ends of the long bones.
3. Important for removing old and defective erythrocytes and platelets from the circulation.
4. Site of haemopoiesis in a fetus at 3 months.
5. Made up of the periarteriolar lymphoid sheath, along with B and T cell follicles.

3. Concerning anaemia:

A. Iron
B. Folate deficiency anaemia
C. Erythrocyte
D. Folate
E. Pernicious anaemia
F. Aplastic anaemia
G. Vitamin B_{12}
H. Sickle cell anaemia
I. Sideroblastic anaemia
J. Iron-deficiency anaemia

Instruction: For each scenario described below, choose the **single** most likely match from the above list of options. Each option may be used once, more than once, or not at all.

1. Anaemia caused by a reduction in number and function of bone marrow stem cells.
2. An anaemia which occurs frequently in women of reproductive age.
3. The Schilling test is used to diagnose the cause of a deficiency of this substance.
4. Anaemia that can present along with chronic atrophic gastritis. Also, probably of autoimmune aetiology.
5. Inherited haemoglobinopathy causing elongation of the red cells into a rigid shape.

4. Concerning clinical presentations of anaemia:

A. Iron deficiency anaemia
B. Anaemia of chronic disease
C. Folate deficiency
D. Pernicious anaemia
E. Sickle cell anaemia
F. Hereditary spherocytosis
G. β-thalassaemia minor
H. Glucose-6-phosphate deficiency (G6PD)
I. Aplastic anaemia
J. Autoimmune haemolytic anaemia

Instruction: For each scenario described below, choose the **single** most likely diagnosis from the above list of options. Each option may be used once, more than once, or not at all.

1. A previously fit and well 26-year-old female is admitted to hospital with a severe dyspnoea, chest pain, productive cough and fever. Her chest radiograph showed patchy consolidation. After several days of admission she begins to improve. The day before her scheduled discharge she suffered from Raynaud's phenomenon. A full blood count showed a megaloblastic anaemia and a direct Coomb's test was positive.
2. A 4-year-old child of African origin presents to Accident and Emergency with a fever and painful, red hands and feet. FBC shows Hb 6.5 g/dL (normal range in children 11–14 g/dL) and mean corpuscular volume (MCV) 100 fL (normal range in children 76–88 fL).
3. A 23-year-old female undergoes a full blood count as part of routine, pre-operative investigations. The results show Hb 10.2 g/dL (normal range for women 12–15 g/dL) and a mean corpuscular volume (MCV) of 71 (normal range 80–100). Further tests reveal a low serum iron, a low ferritin and an increased total iron-binding capacity (TIBC).
4. A 44-year-old man attends his local diabetes clinic. A routine full blood count showed the following: Hb 10.5 g/dL (normal range for men 13–17 g/dL) and a mean corpuscular volume (MCV) 74 fL (normal range 80–100 fL). Iron studies show a low serum iron and a normal total iron-binding capacity (TIBC).
5. A 12-year-old boy from Cyprus becomes jaundiced after a week-long family holiday, where he mainly ate falafel. His full blood count shows a megaloblastic anaemia.

5. Concerning the inheritance of anaemias:

A. β-thalassaemia major
B. β-thalassaemia minor
C. Sickle cell trait
D. Sickle cell anaemia
E. Hereditary spherocytosis
F. Glucose-6-phosphate deficiency
G. Pyruvate kinase deficiency
H. 1 in 4
I. 1 in 2
J. 1 in 16

Instruction: For each scenario described below, choose the **single** most likely match from the above list of options. Each option may be used once, more than once, or not at all.

1. An X-linked disorder, affecting the hexose monophosphate shunt.
2. A rare autosomal recessive condition affecting the glycolytic pathway.
3. An autosomal dominant condition, with variable penetrance. Red cells are less deformable and have increased osmotic fragility.
4. A condition that results from inheriting one defective allele coding for β-chain production.
5. A woman comes to her GP asking advice about planning her family. Her husband has hereditary eliptocytosis. What is the chance that each of her children will be affected?

6. Concerning haematological investigations:

A. Cytogenetic analysis
B. Prothrombin time (PT)
C. Fine needle aspiration
D. Differential white count
E. Erythrocyte sedimentation rate (ESR)
F. Full blood count
G. Serum electrophoresis
H. Bone marrow smear
I. Lymph node biopsy
J. Peripheral blood film

Instruction: For each scenario described below, choose the **single** most likely match from the above list of options. Each option may be used once, more than once, or not at all.

1. Test which allows the examination of different stages of haemopoiesis.
2. The identification of specific levels of neutrophils, lymphocytes, monocytes, eosinophils and basophils in the blood.
3. The rate of fall of a column of red blood cells in plasma over 1 hour.
4. A test to measure the function of the coagulation cascade.
5. The study of the structure and function of chromosomes to highlight any abnormalities which may indicate a certain condition.

7. Concerning white blood cells:

A. B cells
B. Leucopenia
C. Monocytes
D. Neutrophils
E. Natural killer cells
F. T cells
G. Eosinophils
H. Right shift
I. Mast cells
J. Basophils

Instruction: For each scenario described below, choose the **single** most likely match from the above list of options. Each option may be used once, more than once, or not at all.

1. Large, circulating white blood cells, with distinctive, kidney-shaped nuclei.
2. A lymphocyte that matures in the thymus.
3. The first cells recruited to a site of acute inflammation.
4. Cells which mediate the delayed stage in type I hypersensitivity.
5. The appearance of hypersegmented neutrophils in non-infectious inflammatory processes.

8. Concerning haemostasis:

A. Intrinsic pathway
B. Heparin
C. Platelets
D. Fibrin
E. Thrombocytopenia
F. Extrinsic pathway
G. Thrombin
H. Warfarin
I. Vitamin K
J. Anaemia

Instruction: For each scenario described below, choose the **single** most likely match from the above list of options. Each option may be used once, more than once, or not at all.

1. Substance that converts fibrinogen to fibrin in the final stages of the coagulation cascade.
2. Vitamin K antagonist.
3. Process of coagulation which occurs entirely within the circulation.
4. A condition characterized by a decrease in the number of platelets in the blood.
5. The stimulation of the coagulation cascade by tissue factor (TF), a glycoprotein present on fibroblasts.

9. Concerning disorders of haemostasis:

A. Drug induced thrombocytopenia
B. Thrombotic thrombocytopenic purpura
C. von Willebrand's disease
D. Hypersplenism
E. Haemophilia A
F. Haemophilia B
G. Protein C deficiency
H. Disseminated intravascular coagulation
I. Factor V Leiden
J. Antiphospholipid syndrome

Instruction: For each scenario described below, choose the **single** most likely match from the above list of options. Each option may be used once, more than once, or not at all.

1. An immensely dangerous condition that results from excessive activation of the coagulation cascade, followed by activation of the fibrinolytic cascade.
2. An inherited thrombophilia with a 5% prevalence in Caucasians in the UK.
3. An X-linked condition that results in a deficiency of clotting factor IX.
4. The most common bleeding disorder, affecting up to 1% of the population.
5. A condition that results from antibodies to ADAMTS-13.

10. Concerning drugs affecting haemostasis:

A. Warfarin
B. Unfractionated heparin
C. Low-molecular-weight heparin
D. Aspirin
E. Clopidogrel
F. Dipyridamole
G. GPIIb/IIIa inhibitors
H. Streptokinase
I. Urokinase
J. Recombinant tPa

Instruction: For each scenario described below, choose the **single** most likely match from the above list of options. Each option may be used once, more than once, or not at all.

1. A non-specific, irreversible COX inhibitor.
2. A fibrinolytic derived from group A β-haemolytic streptococci.
3. A glycoaminoglycan that potentiated the actions of antithrombin. It is sometimes monitored, using the anti-Xa assay.
4. An ADP receptor antagonist.
5. A vitamin K antagonist.

11. Concerning the management of disorders of haemostasis:

A. Warfarin, with a target INR of 2.5 (2-3).
B. Warfarin, with a target INR of 3 (2.5-3.5).
C. Subcutaneous low-molecular-weight heparin.
D. Intravenous unfractionated heparin.
E. Aspirin.
F. GbIIb/IIIa inhibitor.
G. Recombinant FVIII.
H. Recombinant FIX.
I. Streptokinase.
J. Recombinant tPa.

Instruction: For each scenario described below, choose the **single** most appropriate management from the above list of options. Each option may be used once, more than once, or not at all.

1. A 37-year-old male with haemophilia B presents to Accident and Emergency with a swollen, hot, tender right knee.
2. A 70-year-old obese male presents to Accident and Emergency with chest pain. An ST-elevation myocardial infarction is diagnosed. Primary percutaneous coronary intervention is not available at that hospital. Fibrinolysis is available. He has received fibrinolysis in the past, but the agent is unknown.
3. A 23-year-old pregnant woman is found to have the antiphospholipid antibody syndrome. She already takes aspirin. Once fetal heart activity begins, anticoagulant therapy is indicated.
4. A 65-year-old woman is diagnosed with atrial fibrillation. After considering her risk factors the consultant cardiologist believes that anticoagulant therapy is indicated.
5. A 67-year-old woman suffers a myocardial infarction. She is discharged after recovering well. On discharge she requires a prescription for secondary prevention.

12. Concerning haematological malignancies:

A. Hodgkin's lymphoma
B. Mantle cell lymphoma
C. Follicular lymphoma
D. Acute lymphoblastic leukaemia
E. Acute myeloid leukaemia
F. Chronic lymphocytic leukaemia
G. Chronic myeloid leukaemia
H. Myeloma
I. Waldenström's macroglobulinaemia
J. Myelofibrosis

Instruction: For each scenario described below, choose the **single** most likely match from the above list of options. Each option may be used once, more than once, or not at all.

1. The most common low grade non-Hodgkin's lymphoma.
2. A condition that results from a monoclonal proliferation of plasma cells.
3. A condition characterized by the clonal expansion of lymphoid cells. Reed–Sternberg cells are pathognomonic for this condition.
4. The most common leukaemia in children.
5. A myeloproliferative disorder, often preceded by polycythaemia rubra vera. A dry tap is usually seen in this condition.

13. Concerning the clinical presentation of haematological malignancies:

A. Myelofibrosis
B. Myeloma
C. Hodgkin's lymphoma
D. Chronic lymphocytic leukaemia
E. Mantle cell lymphoma
F. Polycythaemia rubra vera
G. Acute myeloid leukaemia
H. Waldenström's macroglobulinaemia
I. Acute lymphoblastic leukaemia
J. Chronic myeloid leukaemia

Instruction: For each scenario described below, choose the **single** most likely diagnosis from the above list of options. Each option may be used once, more than once, or not at all.

1. A 57-year-old female presents to Accident and Emergency with severe back pain after a fall at home. A back X-ray shows osteolytic lesions with vertebral collapse.
2. A 64-year-old male presents to his GP with fatigue, weight loss, night sweats and a cervical mass. A lymph node biopsy reveals cells that look like 'owl's eyes'.
3. A 53-year-old female presents to her GP with a 4-week history of headache and intermittent dizziness. On examination she looks plethoric and has mild splenomegaly. A full blood count reveals a very high haemoglobin.
4. A 70-year-old female presents to her GP with a persistent sore throat. On direct questioning she admits that she had been feeling more tired than normal recently, but put it down to 'getting old'. A full blood count shows that she has leucopenia. A peripheral blood film demonstrates myeloid blast cells.
5. A 67-year-old male presents to his GP complaining of bone pain and says his vision has been intermittently affected. Serum electrophoresis reveals a monocloncal band of IgM.

14. Concerning the management of haematological malignancies:

A. Tirosine kinase inhibitor (imatinib)
B. Venesection
C. All trans-retinoic acid
D. High-dose chemotherapy and/or radiotherapy
E. Amputation
F. Combination chemotherapy and rituximab
G. Rituximab, cyclophosphamide, doxorubicin, vincristine and prednisolone (R-CHOP)
H. Rituximab alone
I. Hydroxyurea, α-interferon or anagrelide
J. Supportive management, with the possibility of splenectomy

Instruction: For each scenario described below, choose the **single** most appropriate management from the above list of options. Each option may be used once, more than once, or not at all.

1. A 51-year-old female is diagnosed with polycythaemia ruba vera. She has a low thrombotic risk.
2. A 45-year-old male is diagnosed with primary thrombocythaemia. He has a platelet count of 947×10^9/L (normal range 150–400 $\times 10^9$/L).
3. A 65-year-old female is diagnosed with chronic myeloid leukaemia. She is deemed not suitable for a stem cell transplant.
4. A 53-year-old male is diagnosed with diffuse large B-cell lymphoma.
5. A 48-year-old female is diagnosed with acute myeloid leukaemia. Cytogenetic analysis reveals the t(15;17) rearrangement.

15. Concerning blood products:

A. Recombinant factor VIII
B. Cross-matched red cells
C. Platelets
D. Clotting factor VIII concentrate
E. Immunoglobulin
F. Cryoprecipitate
G. Fresh frozen plasma
H. O negative red cells
I. Albumin
J. Intraoperative blood salvage

Instruction: For each scenario described below, choose the **single** most appropriate blood product from the above list of options. Each option may be used once, more than once, or not at all.

1. A 20-year-old male is brought to Accident and Emergency following a serious road traffic collision. His clinical condition is deteriorating and he needs red blood cells immediately. He cannot wait for any blood tests.
2. A 64-year-old male, who has recently been diagnosed with acute myeloid leukaemia, is admitted to a medical ward with breathlessness and fatigue. He is stable but his haemoglobin is 7.7 g/dL (normal range for men 13–17 g/dL).

3. A male Jehovah's witness is scheduled to have a hip replacement. The consultant surgeon discusses blood products with the patient, and the patient makes it clear that he is opposed to receiving all blood products, from others.

4. An 18-year-old boy presents to Accident and Emergency with a 5-hour history of epistaxis. A full blood count reveals a platelet count of 23×10^9/L (normal range 150–400 $\times 10^9$/L).

5. A 28-year-old male with haemophilia A presents to Accident and Emergency with a haematoma in his thigh, after falling over.

16. Concerning complement:

A. Alternative pathway
B. C3
C. Lectin pathway
D. Collectins
E. Anaphylotoxin
F. C1 esterase inhibitor
G. Membrane attack complex
H. C7
I. Classical pathway
J. Complement inhibitors

Instruction: For each scenario described below, choose the **single** most likely match from the above list of options. Each option may be used once, more than once, or not at all.

1. Final set of complement proteins, which form a polymer that punches holes in cell membranes.

2. The initiation of complement proteins by antibodies.

3. Deficient in hereditary angioedema.

4. Causes increased vascular permeability and attracts white blood cells to the site of infection.

5. Regulates the processes involved in the complement cascade.

17. Concerning immunization:

A. Passive immunity
B. Plasma cells
C. Dead vaccine
D. Subunit vaccine
E. Innate immunity
F. Active immunity
G. Memory cells
H. Adjuvant
I. Pathogen
J. Live attenuated vaccine

Instruction: For each scenario described below, choose the **single** most likely match from the above list of options. Each option may be used once, more than once, or not at all.

1. A substance that provides a danger signal to the innate immune system by causing low-grade inflammation.

2. Type of immunity produced as a response to vaccination.

3. Cells which form from clonal expansion of B and T lymphocytes in vaccination, which are activated in a secondary immune response.

4. The transfer of immunoglobulins to an individual.

5. Form of vaccine that requires an adjuvant.

18. Concerning cell surface molecules:

A. B cell receptor
B. Toll-like receptor
C. MHC class I
D. FAS ligand
E. T cell receptor
F. MHC class II
G. Antigen
H. Cell adhesion molecules (CAMs)
I. CD3
J. Collectins

Instruction: For each scenario described below, choose the **single** most likely match from the above list of options. Each option may be used once, more than once, or not at all.

1. Substances recognized by the specific receptors of the adaptive immune system.

2. Pattern recognition molecules found in solution.

3. Molecules which bind and present peptide antigens from intracellular pathogens.

4. Molecule that recognizes intracellular or phagocytosed antigen when it is expressed simultaneously with the major histocompatibility complex (MHC) in which it is lying.

5. Family of related molecules found on cell surfaces which, upon recognizing a pathogen, activate the innate immune system.

19. Concerning immunoglobulins:

A. IgA
B. J-chain
C. Type II hypersensitivity
D. IgM
E. Type I hypersensitivity
F. Type IV hypersensitivity
G. Class switch
H. IgG
I. Type III hypersensitivity
J. Clonal expansion

Instruction: For each scenario described below, choose the **single** most likely match from the above list of options. Each option may be used once, more than once, or not at all.

1. Process by which a single B cell can produce different classes of immunoglobulins.
2. Antibody secreted onto mucosal surfaces.
3. Immune response stimulated by the presence of allergens.
4. Immunoglobulin from which all other immunoglobulins are derived in the process of class switch.
5. Reaction of ABO antigens and antibodies in the blood.

20. Concerning B and T lymphocytes:

A. CD8
B. Myeloid stem cells
C. Plasma cells
D. Basophil
E. Memory B cells
F. T helper cells
G. Cytotoxic T cells
H. Memory T cells
I. CD40
J. Lymphoid stem cells

Instruction: For each scenario described below, choose the **single** most likely match from the above list of options. Each option may be used once, more than once, or not at all.

1. Induces B cells to become fully active and begin releasing antibody.
2. Cells from which B and T lymphocytes originate.
3. Cells with a vast amount of endoplasmic reticulum in order to secrete large quantities of immunoglobulin.
4. Cell marker associated with cytotoxic T cells.
5. Cells which recognize antigen in conjunction with MHC class I.

21. Concerning investigations:

A. Skin prick test.
B. C-reactive protein titre.
C. Enzyme-linked immunosorbent assay (ELISA).
D. Patch test.
E. Polymerase chain reaction (PCR).
F. Flow cytometry.
G. Tuberculin skin test.
H. HLA-typing.
I. Measurement of IgG, IgA and IgM.
J. Differential white cell count.

Instruction: For each scenario described below, choose the **single** most appropriate test from the above list of options. Each option may be used once, more than once, or not at all.

1. The test needed to confirm a primary immunoglobulin deficiency.
2. The test used to measure CD4 counts.
3. The test that involves an intradermal injection of purified protein derivative (PPD).
4. The test that uses radiolabelled antibodies to bind to, and detect, antigens or antigen-antibody complexes.
5. The test used to confirm nickel allergy.

22. Concerning hypersensitivity:

A. Skin prick test
B. Pigeon fancier's disease
C. Post streptococcal glomerulonephritis
D. Nickel allergy
E. Type I hypersensitivity
F. Type III hypersensitivity
G. Atopic eczema
H. ABO incompatibility
I. Type IV hypersensitivity
J. Anaphylaxis

Instruction: For each scenario described below, choose the **single** most likely match from the above list of options. Each option may be used once, more than once, or not at all.

1. A type of hypersensitivity that results from antibody-antigen complex deposition. Farmer's lung is a form of this hypersensitivity.
2. A medical emergency that requires 0.5 mL of 1:1000 of adrenaline intramuscularly as part of the immediate management.
3. A type of hypersensitivity that results from IgE-mediated mast cell degranulation. Allergic rhinitis is a form of this hypersensitivity.
4. A form of type II hypersensitivity.
5. A form of type III hypersensitivity.

---

23. Concerning autoimmunity:

A. Central tolerance
B. Graves' disease
C. Type II diabetes
D. Rheumatoid arthritis
E. Central tolerance
F. Molecular mimicry
G. Systemic lupus erythematosus (SLE)
H. Wegener's granulomatosis
I. Type I diabetes
J. Peripheral tolerance

Instruction: For each scenario described below, choose the **single** most likely match from the above list of options. Each option may be used once, more than once, or not at all.

1. The autoimmune disease caused by the deposition of immune complexes, which often causes a photosensitive rash.
2. The disease which is associated with individuals carrying both HLA-DR3 and HLA-DR4.
3. The immunological process behind rheumatic fever.
4. The process in which self-reactive T cells and B cells are eliminated.
5. A condition that results from stimulatory antibody production.

---

24. Concerning immunological interventions:

A. Non-steroidal anti-inflammatory drugs (NSAIDs)
B. Early referral to a rheumatologist
C. Corticosteroids
D. Adrenaline
E. Interleukin-2 (IL-2) receptor blocker
F. Infliximab
G. Rituximab
H. An allogenic graft
I. C1 inhibitor
J. An autologous graft

Instruction: For each scenario described below, choose the **single** most likely match from the above list of options. Each option may be used once, more than once, or not at all.

1. The 15-year-old son of a patient known to have type I hereditary angioedema presents to Accident and Emergency with breathing difficulty and facial oedema. He has had no contact with potential allergens. He is given a medication intravenously and his clinical state begins to improve.
2. The most appropriate management for a patient with suspected rheumatoid arthritis.
3. A graft between individuals of the same species.
4. A new class of drug that suppresses both T and B cell proliferation and is used to treat transplant rejection.
5. A monoclonal antibody that targets tumour necrosis factor.

---

25. Concerning the immune system in action:

A. Phagocytes
B. Secretory immunoglobin A (sIgA)
C. Tumour necrosis factor alpha (TNF-α)
D. MHC class I
E. Natural killer cells
F. The membrane attack complex (MAC)
G. Mast cells
H. Interferon alpha (IFN-α)
I. Plasma cells
J. Toll-like receptors

Instruction: For each scenario described below, choose the **single** most likely match from the above list of options. Each option may be used once, more than once, or not at all.

1. The cells that release histamine in response to immunoglobulin E stimulation, for example in parasitic infections.
2. The cells that destroy most extracellular bacteria.
3. The cytokine secreted by virally infected cells to communicate with other cells.
4. Viral peptides are presented to CD8 positive T cells by this molecule.
5. The cytokine involved in granuloma formation and maintenance.

MCQ Answers

1. b. Liver and spleen. Refer to sites of haemopoiesis (p. 2) to answer this question.
2. c. Thymus.
3. a. G-CSF. G-CSF acts on the granulocyte precursors helping boost the neutrophil count. Erythropoietin (EPO) stimulates erythrocyte production, while eltrombopag and romiplostim are new therapeutic agents that encourage platelet production. Stem cell factor acts on pluripotent stem cells encouraging their renewal; however, it is not used clinically outside of clinical trials.
4. c. It is encapsulated. All of the above options are true of *Strep. pneumoniae*. However, the spleen is involved in removing encapsulated organisms such as *N. meningitides, Strep. pneumoniae* and *H. influenzae*. Thus, post-splenectomy the patient is more prone to these infections.
5. d. Red marrow is normally restricted to the axial skeleton and the proximal ends of long bones. Red marrow is also where haemopoiesis occurs. Yellow marrow is mainly fat but can become red marrow if the body's haemopoietic demands increase. Haemopoiesis normally occurs in the bone marrow but should the need arise the spleen and the liver can also resume their fetal haemopoietic role. Macrophages are found in the bone marrow and store iron in the form of ferritin and haemosiderin. Red and white pulps are found in the spleen, not the bone marrow.
6. c. They transport CO_2. Erythrocytes are responsible for transporting O_2 and CO_2. They have no nucleus or organelles. Erythrocytes are derived from CFU-GEMM and have an average lifespan of 120 days. They usually have a biconcave discoid shape.
7. d. Primary haemochromatosis is caused by excessive absorption. Primary haemochromatosis is an autosomal recessive condition characterized by excessive absorption of iron. Iron is actively absorbed in the duodenum and jejunum. There is no mechanism to excrete excess iron. Iron is transported in the blood bound to transferrin, it is stored as ferritin when bound to apoferritin. Total body stores are $\sim$4 g4g, and normal daily requirement is $\sim$1 mg.
8. b. Each haemoglobin can carry 4 molecules of oxygen. Adult haemoglobin (HbA) is normally made up of two α-chains and two β-chains. Oxygen binding to haemoglobin follows a sigmoid curve. However, the oxygen dissociation curve of myoglobin is hyperbolic. 2,3-diphosphoglycerate levels rise in hypoxia to allow the release of oxygen to the tissues. The Bohr effect shifts the curve to the right due to an increase in H^+ concentration (a lower pH).
9. a. It may be raised in β-thalassaemia syndromes. This is to compensate for the deficiency in β-chains and therefore defective HbA. Fetal haemoglobin (HbF) is composed of two α and two γ-globin chains, and has a higher affinity of oxygen than HbA. HbF is the primary haemoglobin in the later two-thirds of fetal gestation and up to around 3 months of age. After that levels of HbF should be very low and in adults there is normally $< 1\%$ HbF. 2% of haemoglobin in an adult is HbA_2.
10. e. Unconjugated bilirubin is water insoluble. Haem is produced in the mitochondria of immature red cells, and is broken down by macrophages in the bone marrow, liver and spleen. Haem consists of one Fe^{2+} ion at the centre of a protoporphyrin ring. Bilirubin is conjugated in the liver, making it water soluble. It is then secreted in bile.
11. d. Blood levels of erythropoietin (EPO) are raised at higher altitudes. The major stimulus for EPO secretion is hypoxia, thus at higher altitudes where partial pressures of oxygen are lower EPO levels are raised. Although some EPO originates in the liver the majority ($\sim$90%) comes from the endothelial cells of the peritubular capillaries in the renal cortex. Androgens can increase EPO production but this is not the major stimulus for secretion. Bilateral nephrectomy, rather than splenectomy, decreases EPO production and can cause anaemia.
12. e. Total gastrectomy reduces absorption. Vitamin B_{12} binds to intrinsic factor (which is produced by the parietal cells of the stomach) and is absorbed in the terminal ileum. It is stored in the liver. Vitamin D_3 is synthesized in the skin.
13. c. It is utilized in the metabolism of alcohol. Pernicious anaemia results in deficiency of vitamin B_{12}. Vitamin B_{12} is found exclusively in foods derived from animals (e.g. meat, eggs, milk, fish), whereas folic acid is found mainly in green vegetables, as well as fortified breakfast cereals.
14. b. Renal failure. Normochromic, normocytic anaemias are often caused by chronic disease. Renal failure results in lower levels of the hormone erythropoietin (EPO) and thus, anaemia. Iron deficiency and thalassaemia are most commonly associated with microcytic anaemias. Pernicious anaemia and hereditary spherocytosis are most commonly associated with megaloblastic anaemias.
15. d. Raised serum transferrin. Iron deficiency anaemia can cause brittle nails (koilonychias) rather than

leuconychia, which refers to white nails seen in hypoalbuminaemia. Iron deficiency classically results in microcytic, hypochromic red cells. Ferritin is normally reduced while transferrin (and the total iron-binding capacity) is increased. Subacute combined degeneration of the cord is a serious neurological complication associated with vitamin B_{12} deficiency.

16. d. Low total iron-binding capacity (TIBC). The TIBC is normally raised in iron deficiency anaemia. Both anaemia of chronic disease and iron deficiency anaemia can cause a low haemoglobin, low serum iron and a negative direct Coombs test. The direct Coombs test is normally positive in autoimmune haemolytic anaemias. Although anaemia of chronic disease is normally normocytic, it can also have a microcytic picture, like iron deficiency.

17. d. Jaundice. Haem breakdown results in excess unconjugated bilirubin, and therefore jaundice. Excess bilirubin also results in pigment gall stones, rather than cholesterol gallstones. Glossitis is a feature of iron deficiency, as well as folic acid and vitamin B_{12} deficiency. Haptoglobin is normally decreased in haemolysis, as it binds the free haemoglobin.

18. c. Constipation. Angina can be a symptom of severe anaemia, due to cardiac muscle hypoxia. Peripheral neuropathy is a feature of severe vitamin B_{12} deficiency. Koilonychia is a feature of iron deficiency anaemia. Mouth ulcers are associated with iron and B vitamin deficiencies.

19. b. Endoscopy of the gastrointestinal tract. The blood results suggest iron deficiency anaemia. Iron deficiency anaemia in a man, or a woman past the menopause should prompt investigation for a gastrointestinal (GI) bleed (peptic ulcer or occult GI cancer). Iron deficiency in a woman of childbearing age is most commonly due to menstrual losses.

20. e. Diabetes mellitus is a common complication. In haemochromatosis, iron is deposited in many organs, including the pancreas which leads to diabetes. The skin is often pigmented giving rise to the expression 'bronzed diabetes'. Haemochromatosis occurs after autosomal recessive inheritance of the HFE mutation. There is an excess of iron, rather than a deficiency. Clinical features normally present after the age of 40.

21. b. Low serum folate. This patient appears to have alcohol problems. Alcohol causes folate deficiency because of malabsorption, malnutrition and increased utilization. Iron deficiency anaemia is the most common anaemia in the community, but a macrocytic anaemia makes this unlikely. Vitamin B_{12} also causes a megaloblastic anaemia, however there are large stores in the liver and deficiency is normally caused by pernicious anaemia or intestinal malabsorption. This patient doesn't appear to have either.

22. e. Measure serum folate. Administration of vitamin B_{12} to patients that have folate deficiency can result in the devastating neurological complication subacute combined degeneration of the cord (SCDC). Thus concurrent folate deficiency must be ruled out. Overdoses of vitamin B_{12} are very rare, and mostly harmless, thus initial B_{12} levels are not important. Vitamin B_{12} is safe in pregnancy; in fact increased demand in pregnancy can be the trigger for vitamin B_{12} deficiency, and it responds well to treatment. Vitamin B_{12} is normally given as intramuscular injections and so swallowing difficulties are of no importance.

23. c. Every 3 months.

24. d. Hereditary spherocytosis. This is an autosomal dominant condition which is relatively common in people of Northern European descent. Haemolysis results in a megaloblastic anaemia. Splenectomy is sometimes used to prevent recurrent crises. The cells that appear smaller and thicker in his peripheral blood film are spherocytes.

25. d. The presence of HbA on electrophoresis. Both β-thalassaemia major and minor result in a microcytic, hypochromic anaemia. However, β-thalassaemia minor results in a mild anaemia depending on the mutation. Onset before 9 months of age, skull X-ray changes and splenomegaly are features of β-thalassaemia major. In β-thalassaemia major there is no production of HbA.

26. e. B cells and natural killer (NK) cells tend to be bigger than T cells. Lymphocytes are the smallest white blood cell, with a very large nucleus and few granules. When in the blood, they are only in transit between the bone marrow and lymphoid organs. They are derived from lymphoid stem cells.

27. d. Immature 'band' forms may appear in severe sepsis. This is also known as left shift. Hypersegmented nuclei are seen in right shift, which occurs in non-infectious inflammatory processes. Neutrophils are normally very high in bacterial infections. Neutrophils tend to have a multilobed nucleus, with lots of granules around it. They are normally the most abundant white cell (40–80%).

28. b. Basophils.

29. b. Bone marrow disorders that result in the clonal production of abnormal myeloid cells. a. describes the myeloproliferative disorders, c. describes leukaemias, d. describes lymphomas and e. describes myeloma.

30. d. Chronic myeloid leukaemia. It is also present in a minority of acute lymphoblastic leukaemias, and confers a worse prognosis.

31. e. Myeloma.

32. c. Acute lymphoblastic leukaemia. These signs and symptoms point towards a haematological malignancy. ALL is the most common leukaemia in children and should be ruled out. It is always important to have non-accidental injury in mind when seeing young or vulnerable patients.

33. c. Burkitt's lymphoma. Fatigue, fever and sweating imply a haematological malignancy, most specifically a lymphoma. The age and ethnicity of the patient, coupled with the jaw mass make Burkitt's lymphoma (endemic form) the most likely. A 2-week history makes a sickle cell crisis unlikely.

34. d. Reed–Sternberg cells. This patient appears to be suffering from Hodgkin's lymphoma, which is diagnosed with Reed–Sternberg cells on lymph node biopsy. A pepper-pot skull is seen in myeloma. The Philadelphia chromosome is pathognomonic for chronic myeloid leukaemia (and is sometimes seen in acute lymphoblastic leukaemia). A positive monospot test indicates active Epstein-Barr infection. Having more than 20% myeloid blast cells in the bone marrow is indicative of acute myeloid leukaemia.

35. a. Primary polycythaemia.

36. d. Trephine biopsy.

37. c. It is associated with pathological arthrodesis. Inheritance is X-linked and it is unrelated to social class. Haemophilia A is caused by factor VIII deficiency. Factor IX deficiency is haemophilia B. Epistaxis is a common feature of platelet disorders, as opposed to joint and muscle bleeds which are more common in haemophilias.

38. b. The coagulation cascade culminates in thrombin cleaving fibrinogen into fibrin. The FIXa-FVIIIa-Ca^{2+} is the tenase complex which is a potent activator of FX. Prothrombin is cleaved by the prothrombinase complex (FXa-FVa-Ca^{2+}). The APTT measure the intrinsic pathway, while the prothrombin time (PT) assesses the extrinsic pathway. The surface of platelets is integral to the propagation step of haemostasis. Protein S is a cofactor in the inactivation of FVa and FVIIIa.

39. e. Warfarin therapy. Warfarin affects the vitamin K-dependent clotting factors (II,VII, IX and X) and mainly affects the extrinsic pathway. The extrinsic pathway is measured with the prothrombin time (PT). Warfarin therapy is monitored using the international normalised ratio (INR) which comes from the PT. Haemophilias A and B (deficiency of factors VIII and IX respectively) effect the intrinsic pathway and therefore have prolonged activated partial thromboplastin times (APTT). von Willebrand's disease affects platelets and therefore would most likely affect the bleeding time, rather than the clotting times (although it may cause a mild prolongation of the APTT). Protein C deficiency would decrease the PT rather than prolong it.

40. c. Warfarin is teratogenic. For this reason anticoagulation during pregnancy should be in the form of heparin, which doesn't cross the placenta. Warfarin affects the extrinsic pathway and hence is measured using the prothrombin time and international normalised ratio (INR). A lower INR means a lower prothrombin time, and therefore more risk of clotting. The half-life of warfarin is approximately 40 hours, so its effects take around 2 days to wear off. Warfarin often interacts with other medications, and therefore bleeding risk is affected. Patients on warfarin should consult their doctor or pharmacist before starting any new medication (including over-the-counter or herbal remedies).

41. c. It irreversibly inhibits cyclo-oxygenase. a. describes the mechanism of clopidogrel. c. describes how dipyridamole works. e. describes warfarin.

42. d. Atrial fibrillation (AF). AF is associated with thrombotic risk and most patients with AF are anticoagulated with warfarin or aspirin. The other answers are associated with an increased risk of bleeding.

43. b. Prothrombin. The vitamin K-dependent clotting factors are factors II (prothrombin), VII, IX and X.

44. e. anti-Xa assay.

45. d. A couple who are both blood group O will only have group O children. The blood group O gene is recessive to both A and B genes. The most common blood group is O. People who are blood group AB will be self-tolerant to both A and B red cell antigens and so will have no A or B antibodies. Anti-A and anti-B antibodies are normally IgM. Group O plasma contains anti-A and anti-B antibodies, and so can only be given to patients with blood group O.

46. a. All anti-D antibodies are IgG. ~85% of Caucasians are Rh D positive. Anti-D antibodies are acquired after sensitization (alloimmunization) e.g. transfusion of Rh D positive blood. The D antigen is the strongest immunogen of all the Rh antigens. Rh D positive individuals have one or two D alleles (i.e. their genotype is Dd or DD). If both parents have a Dd genotype there is a one in four chance that their child will not inherit a D allele. Their genotype would therefore be dd, making them Rh D negative.

47. d. Anti-D antibody should be given to all rhesus D negative mothers during pregnancy. HDN is most commonly caused by rhesus D incompatibility, but not exclusively. Other forms of incompatibility (e.g. ABO) can occur. Rhesus negative mothers require a sensitizing experience to create their own anti-D antibodies. Thus it normally happens with pregnancies after carrying a rhesus positive child. Rhesus D antibodies are always IgG. HDN is very serious and often results in hydrops fetalis.

48. c. Low back pain.

49. b. Factor VIII.

50. b. Fresh frozen plasma. This patient has received a massive transfusion. Red cells are deficient in clotting factors (specifically factors V and VIII), as well as platelets. The blood results from the question indicate that she has a coagulopathy. The only answer from those available that would replace her clotting factors is fresh frozen plasma.

51. c. It is composed of phagocytes and complement. The other answers describe the adaptive immune system.

52. d. CD4+ T lymphocytes recognize antigen associated with MHC class II. Antibodies are produced by plasma cells. T helper cells are normally CD4+. CD8+ T cells are not phagocytes, but can destroy cells using other methods.

53. c. IgA. IgA is present in high concentrations in colostrum. It coats the mucosal surfaces of the gastrointestinal tract and affords some protection from pathogens while the immune system develops.

54. a. Macrophage.

55. b. Lysosome.

56. e. Neutrophils.

57. d. Natural killer cells. CD8+ T cells can also carry out this function.

58. b. C-reactive protein. C-reactive protein (CRP) is an important marker of inflammation used clinically to assess inflammation and monitor response to treatment. The other options are all cytokines.

59. d. Antigen-antibody complexes activate C1. a. describes the alternative pathway, while c. describes the lectin pathway. b. Describes the activation of B cells. e. Describes the activation of cytotoxic T cells.

60. d. C3b. Macrophages have a C3b receptor allowing the opsonization of some bacteria. C3a and C5a are responsible for recruiting phagocytes, as well as degranulation of mast cells. C1 is activated during the classical pathway.

61. c. Osmotic lysis. The membrane attack complex (MAC), made up of C5b-C6-C7-C8-C9, punches a hole in the pathogen's cell membrane, allowing water to rush in and destroy the pathogen.

62. c. C1 inhibitor deficiency.

63. b. The haplotype is found on chromosome 6.

64. e. Class switching. Somatic hypermutation and affinity maturation are different names for the same process that increases the affinity of an antibody for its antigen. Junctional diversity refers to the increased variability in antibodies due to the formation of junctions between the various gene segments. Positive selection refers to the process in which T cells that are able to recognize self-MHC survive, whereas those that cannot do not.

65. a. IgM.

66. c. Somatic hypermutation of immunoglobulin genes occurs in the germinal centres. B cells are activated in the follicles of secondary lymphoid organs. The expression of bcl-2 prevents apoptosis of the B-cell. B cells are activated after dendritic cells present antigen. Activated T helper cells aid B cells in producing antibody by producing cytokines.

67. d. IgE.

68. a. IgG. IgM, on the other hand, is the main immunoglobulin involved in the primary immune response.

69. b. It begins to reduce in size after puberty. The embryonic thymus develops from the third pharyngeal pouch. It is located in the anterior part of the superior mediastinum and has two lobes. A small minority of thymocytes mature and they leave the thymus from the medulla via the postcapillary venules.

70. c. DiGeorge syndrome. Down, Edwards' and Patau's syndromes are all caused by trisomies (21, 18 and 13 respectively). Graves' disease is an autoimmune disease of the thyroid.

71. b. Staphylococcal enterotoxin. Toxic shock syndrome is a very dangerous condition requiring prompt fluid resuscitation and antibiotic therapy.

72. c. Homing due to integrin molecules. Histamine is normally one of the chemical mediators released in acute inflammation, along with cytokines and chemokines. There is usually local vasodilatation (hence redness and heat) with increased vascular permeability, which leads to an inflammatory exudate and therefore swelling. Leucocytes leave the blood and enter the tissues.

73. d. Peyer's patches. Other examples include the pharyngeal tonsils and the appendix.

74. d. The heavy chain determines the class of immunoglobulin. There are two Fab fragments and just one Fc fragment. The N terminal of the light chain is variable while the C terminal is constant.

75. a. Antibodies can neutralize virus particles, as well as act as an opsonin against virally infected cells. Interferon gamma activates macrophages and natural killer cells. Viral peptides are presented on class I MHC molecules. The class I MHC molecules bind to CD8+ T cells enabling them to destroy infected cells. e. describes the actions of CD4+ T helper cells.

76. a. Being a latent virus.

77. e. Secretory immunoglobulin A (sIgA). sIgA can bind to bacteria and prevent them from binding to epithelial cells.

78. d. They have a lipid bilayer. This is the only characteristic above that is particular to Gram-negative bacteria. The MAC can perforate the lipid bilayer and cause osmotic lysis.

79. e. Phagocytes.

80. b. Protozoa have complex life cycles which present the immune system with a variety of challenges.

81. d. Eosinophils.

82. c. Allergic rhinitis. IgE-mediated degranulation of mast cells is the cause of type I hypersensitivity reactions.

83. a. Skin prick testing. A small amount of the allergen is injected into the skin. The response is compared to a histamine control.

84. b. Farmer's lung. Type III hypersensitivity is due to immune complex deposition.

85. e. T helper cells. These cells secrete cytokines on contact with the antigen resulting in the attraction and activation of macrophages. This process takes 24–72 hours to peak, hence the name delayed-type hypersensitivity.

86. d. IM adrenaline (0.5 mL of 1:1000). This dose is one that should be known by all medical professionals. a. b. and c. are all used but later on in the management. C1 inhibitor is used in hereditary angioedema.

87. c. Myasthenia gravis. This disease is characterized by muscle weakness and fatigability.

88. b. Coeliac disease. The anti-tissue transglutaminase test is very sensitive and specific for coeliac disease but confirmation is needed with a duodenal biopsy.

89. b. Rheumatoid arthritis. Type IV autoimmune diseases are characterized by autoimmune T cells responses. Contact dermatitis is a form of type IV hypersensitivity, but is not autoimmune in nature.

90. b. Tumour necrosis factor alpha. TNF-α is important for the infiltration of mononuclear cells and is the target of newer disease modifying anti-rheumatic drugs.

91. a. IgM anti-IgG antibodies. Rheumatoid factor is positive in approximately 75% of patients.

92. c. Acquired immunodeficiency syndrome. The rest are forms of primary immunodeficiency.

93. c. A single-stranded RNA retrovirus. HIV possesses reverse transcriptase with allows it to manufacture double-stranded DNA which is incorporated into host cells genetic material.

94. d. gp120. Once gp120 binds to the CD4 and CCR5 receptor a conformational change results in the expression of gp 41, which allows the virus to enter the cell.

95. b. Bacille Calmette-Guérin. This vaccine immunizes against tuberculosis. Live attenuated vaccines are alive but with a reduced virulence. They should never be given to immunocompromised patients.

96. d. Live attenuated vaccines produce a good cell-mediated response. Vaccines should be immunogenic if they are going to stimulate a host response. The MMR vaccines are live attenuated vaccines. Live attenuated vaccines are more expensive than killed vaccines, and can rarely induce disease in the immunocompromised.

97. e. Acute cellular response takes several days to develop. Hyperacute rejection is rapid because antibodies have been induced prior to transplantation e.g. by blood transfusion. It is prevented by cross-matching the donor cells and recipient serum. Chronic rejection is not well understood and if it occurs, it cannot be treated. Acute cellular rejection is mediated by T cells (as it is type IV hypersensitivity reaction).

98. d. Interleukin-2 receptor. IL-2 is the growth factor for all lymphocytes, therefore blocking the receptor causes severe immunosuppression.

99. b. Gastritis. Inhibition of COX-1 decreases gastroprotective prostaglandins, resulting in increased stomach acid production. This can cause gastritis and peptic ulcers. COX-1 blockade also reduces platelet aggregation, hence aspirin is used as an antiplatelet agent. Cushing's syndrome and osteoporosis are important adverse effects of corticosteroid therapy. Non-steroidal anti-inflammatory drugs (NSAIDs) have antipyretic and analgesic properties as well as their actions against inflammation.

100. e. Non-steroidal anti-inflammatory drugs (NSAIDs) may be nephrotoxic and cause bronchospasm. NSAIDs act by inhibiting the COX enzymes. Hydrocortisone is given intravenously or topically. Oral preparations of corticosteroids come in the form of prednisolone. Paracetamol is not a good anti-inflammatory but is a good antipyretic and analgesic. The gastrointestinal side-effects of NSAIDs are mediated by COX-1 blockade.

EMQ Answers

1. Concerning red blood cells:

1. E. Erythropoietin is a highly glycosylated polypeptide hormone. Its stimulation causes the differentiation and maturation of erythrocytes.
2. A. Red blood cells contain a red pigment, haemoglobin, which binds and transports oxygen and carbon dioxide. It is composed of two α-chains, with either two β- or two δ-chains.
3. C. The breakdown of red blood cells by macrophages produces bilirubin, which is conjugated in the liver and then excreted in bile.
4. I. Immature red blood cells present in the bone marrow and bloodstream are termed reticulocytes.
5. B. Erythropoiesis is the process by which red blood cells are produced in the bone marrow.

2. Concerning the spleen and bone marrow:

1. I. Macrophages are important for the storage of iron in the bone marrow.
2. C. Red marrow is the site of haemopoiesis and is normally restrictced to the axial skeleton and the proximal ends of long bones.
3. G. The red pulp of the spleen forms part of the reticuloendothelial system (RES). The RES is important for removing old and effective red cells and platelets.
4. B. Before 6 weeks' gestation the fetal yolk sac is most important. Between 6 weeks and 6 months the fetal liver and spleen take over.
5. H. The white pulp of the spleen is made up of the periarteriolar lymphoid sheath, along with B and T cell follicles.

3. Concerning anaemia:

1. F. Aplastic anaemia arises from a reduction in the number and function of bone marrow stem cells.
2. J. Iron-deficiency anaemia occurs frequently in women of reproductive age as iron is lost during menstruation as a component of haemoglobin, the red pigment found in red blood cells.
3. G. The cause of vitamin B_{12} deficiency can be diagnosed using the Schilling test.
4. E. Pernicious anaemia can present as chronic atrophic gastritis; it has a probable autoimmune aetiology.
5. H. Sickle cell anaemia is an inherited condition in which red blood cells become elongated into a rigid shape.

4. Concerning clinical presentations of anaemia:

1. J. The macrocytic anaemia and the positive direct Coomb's test point towards an autoimmune haemolysis. This patient is suffering from an atypical pneumonia probably caused by *Mycoplasma pneumonia*, which triggered the haemolysis.
2. E. The presentation sounds like hand-foot syndrome, thought to be caused by sickled red cells occluding the small vessels of the hands and feet.
3. A. The laboratory results suggest iron deficiency anaemia. This is very common, especially in woman of child-bearing age.
4. B. Anaemia of chronic disease can be caused by many chronic conditions including diabetes, obesity, neoplasms and chronic inflammatory conditions.
5. H. Haemolysis can be triggered by fava beans in the Mediterranean type of G6PD.

5. Concerning the inheritance of anaemias:

1. F. Of the 400 variants of glucose-6-phosphate deficiency the two most common are the African and Mediterranean types.
2. G. The disruption to the glycolytic pathway results in a lack of ATP production.
3. E. Spherocytes are also seen on the peripheral blood film. It results from a defective cytoskeleton protein, most commonly spectrin.
4. B. Often known as β-thalassaemia trait. Patients are normally asymptomatic.
5. I. Hereditary elliptocytosis is autosomal dominant thus each child has a 1 in 2 chance of inheriting the affected allele.

6. Concerning haematological investigations:

1. H. The different stages of haemopoiesis can be seen by analysis of a bone marrow smear.
2. D. A differential white count identifies specific levels of neutrophils, lymphocytes, monocytes, eosinophils and basophils in the blood.
3. E. Erythrocyte sedimentation rate (ESR) measures the rate of fall of a column of red blood cells in plasma over 1 hour.
4. B. The function of the coagulation cascade can be assessed by measuring the prothrombin time (PT), a measure of the time it takes for blood to clot.
5. A. Cytogenetic analysis involves the study of the structure and function of chromosomes. This allows any abnormalities to be highlighted and hence can lead to the diagnosis of certain conditions.

7. Concerning white blood cells:

1. C. Monocytes are precursors of macrophages; they are large, circulating white blood cells, with distinctive, kidney-shaped nuclei.
2. F. Lymphoid progenitor cells mature in the thymus to become T cells.
3. D. The first cells recruited to a site of acute inflammation are neutrophils, which are drawn to the area by chemotaxis.
4. G. The delayed stage of type I hypersensitivity is mediated by eosinophils.
5. H. These non-infectious inflammatory processes include malignancy, megaloblastic anaemia, iron deficiency, liver disease, uraemia.

8. Concerning haemostasis:

1. G. Thrombin is an enzyme present during the final stages of the coagulation cascade; it converts fibrinogen to fibrin.
2. H. Warfarin is a vitamin K antagonist and therefore inhibits blood clotting.
3. A. The intrinsic clotting pathway takes place entirely within the bloodstream.
4. E. Thrombocytopenia is a decrease in the number of platelets in the blood, resulting in a decreased ability to clot and the potential for increased bleeding.
5. F. The extrinsic clotting pathway is stimulated by tissue factor (TF), a glycoprotein present on fibroblasts.

9. Concerning disorders of haemostasis:

1. H. This condition is not fully understood. Early diagnosis and intervention are required for a chance of preventing almost certain mortality.
2. I. Caused by a missense mutation of the gene coding for clotting factor V.
3. F. Also known as Christmas disease.
4. C. This is caused by either a deficiency or a defect in von Willebrand's factor (vWF).
5. B. It commonly affects young adults and causes fever, haemolysis and renal failure.

10. Concerning drugs affecting haemostasis:

1. D. Used in secondary prevention of cardiovascular disease.
2. H. It is highly antigenic. Patients will develop antibodies against it, and so subsequent administration can result in an anaphylactic reaction.
3. C. Low-molecular-weight heparin (LMWH) is often used in pregnancy, as it doesn't cross the placenta. It should be monitored using the anti-Xa assay.
4. E. Clopidogrel is used in the acute management of acute coronary syndromes, with aspirin.
5. A. Warfarin is widely used and is monitored using the international normalised ratio (INR).

11. Concerning the management of disorders of haemostasis:

1. H. This patient has a haemoarthrosis. He requires recombinant FIX replacement.
2. J. Fibrinolysis is indicated in ST-elevation myocardial infarctions, if primary percutaneous coronary intervention is not available. Given he may have received streptokinase in the past; the only safe option is recombinant tPa.
3. C. Low-molecular-weight heparin (LMWH) is safe in pregnancy, as it doesn't cross the placenta. This is unlike warfarin, which is teratogenic.
4. A. The international normalized ratio (INR) should be monitored regularly and the patient should consult a doctor (or a pharmacist) before starting any new medications.
5. E. Secondary prevention after a myocardial infarction involves aspirin, and ACE-inhibitor, a β-blocker and a statin. In aspirin hypersensitivity clopidogrel is

indicated instead. In certain circumstances clopidogrel is indicated as well as aspirin.

12. Concerning haematological malignancies:

1. C. Follicular lymphoma is the most common low-grade lymphoma. Management depends on the stage.
2. H. The malignant proliferation of plasma cells results in a monoclonal paraprotein and/or light chain.
3. A. Hodgkin's lymphoma often presents with non-tender lymphadenopathy, especially affecting the cervical and axillary lymph nodes.
4. D. 80% of leukaemias in children are acute lymphoblastic leukaemia. It is associated with other conditions such as Down syndrome.
5. J. Myelofibrosis is characterized by a proliferation of pluripotent stem cells, and the bone marrow is replaced by fibrosis. This fibrosis causes the dry tap.

13. Concerning the clinical presentation of haematological malignancies:

1. B. Osteolytic lesions can cause pathological fractures. Localized bone pain in general should raise suspicions of myeloma.
2. C. 'Owl's eyes' seen on lymph node biopsy refers to Reed–Sternberg cells. There is a bimodal incidence of Hodgkin's lymphoma.
3. F. The symptoms of polycythaemia rubra vera can be attributed to hyperviscosity. Pruritus, made worse by hot showers or baths, is also a common feature.
4. G. A bone marrow sample demonstrating $>$ 20% blasts cells would confirm the diagnosis.
5. B. Management for symptomatic patients includes chemotherapy and rituximab.

14. Concerning the management of haematological malignancies:

1. B. Venesection is a simple way of reducing the packed cell volume. If she had a high thrombotic risk cytotoxic drugs or radiotherapy may be indicated.
2. I. Hydroxycarbamide, α-interferon and anagrelide are effective at reducing platelet counts.
3. A. Tirosine kinase inhibitors are first line for treating chronic myeloid leukaemia. In those who are fit enough stem cell transplant is potentially curative.
4. G. R-CHOP is an effective combination in the management of high-grade lymphomas, such as diffuse large B-cell lymphoma.
5. C. t(15;17) is associated with acute promyelocytic leukaemia and is the only form of acute myeloid leukemia (AML) which responds to all trans-retinoic acid.

15. Concerning blood products:

1. H. If a cross-match cannot be performed the only safe option is O negative red cells.
2. B. The safest way of giving red cells, if there is time, is to give cross-matched red cells.
3. J. The religious beliefs and convictions of the patient should always be taken into consideration, to maintain the patient's autonomy. Intraoperative blood salvage is an acceptable alternative for some, but should be discussed fully to get informed consent.
4. C. This patient is thrombopenic and requires platelets to arrest the bleeding.
5. A. Recombinant factor VIII is now preferable to factor VIII concentrate, in the UK.

16. Concerning complement:

1. G. The membrane attack complex is a set of complement proteins which, on stimulation of the complement cascade, form a polymer that destroys pathogens by punching holes in the cell membrane.
2. I. The classical pathway is a rapid complement activation pathway, initiated by the presence of antibody.
3. F. C1 esterase inhibitor is deficient in patients with hereditary angioedema.
4. E. Anaphylotoxin stimulates the release of histamine, which causes increased vascular permeability and attracts white blood cells to the site of infection.
5. J. The processes involved in the complement cascade are regulated by complement inhibitors.

17. Concerning immunization:

1. H. An adjuvant is a substance added to vaccines which provides a danger signal to the innate immune system through the stimulation of low-grade inflammation.
2. F. Active immunity is an immune response produced by the presence of antigen in vaccines.

3. G. Clonal expansion of B and T lymphocytes in vaccination produces memory cells, which are activated in a secondary immune response. As a result, the secondary immune response is stronger, occurs faster and lasts longer than the primary.
4. A. The transfer of immunoglobulin from one individual to another is termed passive immunity.
5. D. A subunit vaccine requires an adjuvant to improve the immune response.

18. Concerning cell surface molecules:

1. G. Antigens are substances specifically recognized by receptors of the adaptive immune system.
2. J. Collectins are a family of pattern recognition molecules that recognize and opsonize pathogens in solution.
3. C. Major histocompatibility complex (MHC) class I recognizes antigen from intracellular pathogens.
4. E. Intracellular or phagocytosed antigens expressed simultaneously with MHC are recognized by the T cell receptor on the surface of T lymphocytes.
5. B. Toll-like receptors are a family of related molecules found on mammalian cell surfaces; they activate the innate immune system after exposure to a pathogen.

19. Concerning immunoglobulins:

1. G. Class switch allows different types of immunoglobulin to be produced by individual B cells. During class switch, the heavy chains are switched while retaining the same variable chain.
2. A. IgA is an immunoglobulin which is adapted to be secreted across mucosal surfaces.
3. E. Type I hypersensitivity is the immune response stimulated by the presence of allergens, a process mediated by IgE.
4. D. During class switch, all immunoglobulins are derived from molecules of IgM produced by B lymphocytes.
5. C. The reaction of ABO antigens and antibodies in the bloodstream is type II hypersensitivity.

20. Concerning B and T lymphocytes:

1. F. In order to become fully active and begin releasing antibody, B cells must be stimulated by T helper cells.
2. J. B and T cells originate from lymphoid stem cells in the bone marrow.
3. C. Plasma cells are a mature type of B lymphocyte. They contain vast amounts of endoplasmic reticulum in order to produce a large quantity of immunoglobulin.
4. A. CD8 is a cell surface marker expressed on cytotoxic T cells.
5. G. Cytotoxic T cells recognize antigen in conjunction with molecules of major histocompatibility complex (MHC) class I.

21. Concerning investigations:

1. I. This test measures the levels of immunoglobulin.
2. F. Patients with HIV should have their CD4 counts measured, at least, every 3–6 months.
3. G. This test measures previous exposure to *M. tuberculosis* or the bacille Calmette-Guérin (BCG) vaccine. Previous exposure to either results in a firm, red lesion at the site of injection 48–72 hours later. It is caused by infiltration of macrophages and T cells. The tuberculin skin test is being superseded by blood test, including gamma interferon release assays (IGRA).
4. C. This test is used extensively in medicine. It is used to detect antibodies such as in detecting anti-HIV antibodies.
5. D. Nickel allergy is a delayed type (IV) hypersensitivity reaction. Patch testing is used to diagnose this type of hypersensitivity. As opposed to skin prick testing which is used in type I hypersensitivity.

22. Concerning hypersensitivity:

1. F. This hypersensitivity is as a result of soluble antigen and antibody interactions.
2. J. All patients with a suspected or proven case of anaphylaxis should be seen by a specialist in allergy clinic.
3. E. Allergic rhinitis, also known as 'hay fever', causes considerable morbidity to individuals. Management includes antihistamines and local (intranasal) corticosteroids.
4. H. Other forms of type II hypersensitivity include haemolytic disease of the newborn and autoimmune haemolytic anaemia.
5. C. Occurs following a group A beta haemolytic streptococcal infection of the throat or the skin (impetigo).

23. Concerning autoimmunity:

1. G. Most patients with systemic lupus erythematosus (SLE) have antibodies against double-stranded DNA.
2. I. Type I diabetes is caused by destruction of β-cells in the islets of Langerhans.
3. F. The antibodies made against (group A) Streptococcal antigens cross-react with cardiac muscle.
4. E. This negative selection occurs in the thymus for T cells and in the bone marrow for B cells.
5. B. The antibodies stimulated the thyroid stimulating hormone (TSH) receptor, resulting in hyperthyroidism.

24. Concerning immunological interventions:

1. I. This autosomal dominant condition presents with swellings.
2. B. Individuals with rheumatoid arthritis should be referred to a rheumatologist early to commence non-steroidal anti-inflammatory drugs (NSAIDs), disease-modifying anti-rheumatic drugs (DMARDs) and steroids.
3. H. An autologous graft comes from the same person. If a graft comes from a different species it is known as a xenograft, e.g. porcine heart valves.
4. E. IL-2 receptor blockers are potent immunosuppressants and are only used to treat rejection, rather than to prevent it.
5. F. Infliximab is used in conditions such as rheumatoid arthritis.

25. Concerning the immune system in action:

1. G. This response is also the basis of type I hypersensitivity.
2. A. Phagocytes destroy most extracellular bacteria with the help of C3b and antibody.
3. H. IFN-α (and -β) inhibit transcription and translation of viral proteins in neighbouring cells.
4. D. Class I major histocompatibility complex (MHC) molecule present intracellular antigens to CD8+ T cells.
5. C. Granulomas typically appear as an accumulation of lymphocytes and macrophages around a central area of caseous necrosis.

Glossary

Active immunity Resistance to an infection or disease which develops as a result of infection or vaccination.

Adaptive immunity An immune response which is slow to respond, producing lasting immunity which can be humoral or cell mediated.

Adjuvant Substance which enhances the immune response to a vaccine.

Agglutination The process by which suspended bacteria, cells or particles clump together.

Allergen Antigenic substance which stimulates a hypersensitivity reaction.

ANCA Antinuclear cytoplasmic antibody, antibodies directed against proteinase-3 (cANCA) or against myeloperoxidase (pANCA).

Antibody Protein produced by B lymphocytes in response to the presence of an antigen.

Antigen Molecules which are recognized specifically by receptors on cells of the adaptive immune system.

Antigen-presenting cells Cells capable of presenting antigenic material to cells of the adaptive immune system.

Autoimmunity When the body's own defences are targeted against normal body cells.

Apoptosis Programmed cell death.

Atopy Possessing a genetic predisposition to an allergy.

Chemotaxis The movement of cells in response to chemicals, often to a site of infection.

Collectins A family of pattern recognition molecules, present in solution, which stimulate the innate immune system in response to a pathogen.

Complement A series of enzymatic reactions stimulated by the presence of a pathogen.

Cytokine Intercellular molecules used to transmit messages from one cell to another.

Degranulation The release of the preformed secretory granule contents by fusion with the plasma membrane.

Ecchymoses (bruises) Diffuse flat haemorrhages under the skin.

Erythropoietin A hormone, secreted by the kidney, which regulates erythropoiesis.

Haemorrhage Loss of circulating blood.

Haematocrit The relative volume of erythrocytes in the blood.

Haematoma Distinct local swelling caused by loss of blood into a muscle or subcutaneous tissue.

Haptens Small molecules which need to be bound to a large carrier molecule to be immunogenic.

HLA Human leucocyte antigen, the human form of MHC. Cell surface proteins that present antigen.

Hypersensitivity The inappropriate response of the immune system to an antigen.

Immunity A state of relative resistance to a disease.

Immunoglobulin (Ig) A protein substance secreted from plasma cells in response to infection.

Inflammation Localized response to tissue damage characterized by redness, swelling, pain, oedema and increased white cell count.

Interferon A cytokine which is targeted against viruses and intracellular bacteria.

Innate immune system Produces a non-specific response to an infection or disease.

MHC Major histocompatibility complex, a cluster of genes encoding for cell surface receptors which express antigen on the surface of cells.

Opsonin Substance that binds to a molecule to enhance its uptake by a phagocyte.

Passive immunity Passage of immunity from one individual to another.

Pathogen An organism that causes disease.

Pattern recognition molecules Molecules present either in solution or on the surface of cells which are capable of recognizing molecules characteristic of infection.

PCV Packed cell volume, measure of the proportion of blood occupied by red blood cells.

Petechiae Punctuate haemorrhages <2 mm in diameter, usually clustered.

Polymorphism Slight differences in the genetic material of individuals within a population.

Purpura Any condition with bleeding into the skin or mucous membrane.

Toll-like receptor Family of pattern recognition molecules on the cell surfaces which stimulate the innate immune system in response to a pathogen.

Urticaria Also called hives or nettle rash, characterized by an area of red inflammation and raised white bumps.

Vertical transmission Transmission of an infection from mother to fetus.

Vaccine A suspension of antigenic material injected to produce immunity against infection and disease.

Index

Note: Page numbers followed by *b* indicate boxes, *f* indicate figures and *t* indicate tables.

I

J

K

L

M

N

O

P

R

S

T

U

V

W

X